ADVANCES IN HEALTH AND DISEASE

VOLUME 14

ADVANCES IN HEALTH AND DISEASE

Additional books and e-books in this series can be found on Nova's website under the Series tab.

ADVANCES IN HEALTH AND DISEASE

VOLUME 14

LOWELL T. DUNCAN
EDITOR

nova
Medicine & Health
New York

Library of Congress Cataloging-in-Publication Data

ISBN: 978-1-53616-380-3

Published by Nova Science Publishers, Inc. † New York

CONTENTS

Preface		**vii**
Chapter 1	Zika Virus Infection: A New Thread for Pregnancy *Ciro Comparetto and Franco Borruto*	**1**
Chapter 2	Multiple Myeloma: Biological Characteristics, Clinical Aspects and Therapeutic Approaches *Sara Grammatico and Maria Teresa Petrucci*	**115**
Chapter 3	Hyperbaric Oxygen Therapy in Sudden Sensorineural Hearing Loss *Sema Zer Toros, Omer Cagatay Ertugay and Cigdem Kalaycik Ertugay*	**147**
Chapter 4	Secondary, Off-Label Uses of Ruxolitinib *Julia Song, Alice Song, Trisa Palmares, Michael Song and Harold Song*	**155**
Chapter 5	Adverse Health Effects of Benzene Exposure in Children: Current Understandings and Perspectives *Mark A. D'Andrea and G. Kesava Reddy*	**165**

Chapter 6 Prediction of Aquatic Toxicity in Pimephales Promelas of Substituted Benzenes in Silico Methodologies **187**
Nadia Ziani, Khadidja Amirat and Djelloul Messadi

Contents of Earlier Volumes **201**

Index **209**

PREFACE

Advances in Health and Disease. Volume 14 opens with a chapter on Zika Virus, a ribonucleic acid virus of the Flaviviridae family, genus Flavivirus, Spondweni group, Zika species, isolated for the first time in 1947 from a primate in the Zika Forest in Uganda, a natural reserve near Entebbe.

Next, the authors discuss multiple myeloma, which is characterized by the expansion of monoclonal plasma cells in the bone marrow. In about 95% of cases, the aberrant plasma cells produce a monoclonal immunoglobulin called monoclonal component that can be considered a marker of the disease.

Hyperbaric oxygen therapy is explored in the context of sudden sensorineural hearing loss, where it has been used as a treatment since 1979. This exposes a patient to 100% oxygen at a pressure level higher than 1 atmosphere absolute in a specially designed sealed chamber. This facilitates a delivery of increased partial pressure of oxygen to the tissues.

The authors discuss off-label uses of ruxolitinib, particularly in the treatment of myelofibrosis and polycythemia vera, as drugs can sometimes have uses beyond the official approved indication.

Following this, summaries of the current scientific knowledge and understanding of the clinical findings and health consequences of benzene exposure among children are presented. Children at various developmental stages have unique physical risk factors when exposed to toxic chemicals such as benzene due to their levels of mobility, oxygen consumption, hormonal production, and overall growth.

Lastly, a hybrid quantitative structure–activity relationship model was developed for the prediction of aqueous toxicity. The data concerning 92 substituted benzenes was separated into two disjoined subsets, respectively 74 elements for calculating and testing of the model, and 18 elements for its external validation.

Chapter 1 - Zika Virus (ZIKV) is a ribonucleic acid (RNA) virus of the *Flaviviridae* family, genus *Flavivirus*, *Spondweni* group, *Zika* species, isolated for the first time in 1947 from a primate in Uganda, in the Zika Forest, a natural reserve near Entebbe. In the years 2010, there were occurrences of the disease in all continents and isolated cases were also recorded in Europe, on subjects who were returning from travel in tropical areas and without any form of transmission of the virus in Europe. In humans, it causes a disease known as "zika" or zika fever. The virus is closely related to those that cause dengue, yellow fever, West Nile encephalitis, and Japanese encephalitis, all transmitted mainly by insect bites and therefore called "arthropode-borne viruses" (arboviruses). The virus is transmitted by numerous mosquitoes of the genus *Aedes*, in equatorial environments especially by *Aedes aegypti*. Studies on the vectors involved in the transmission of the virus have allowed to isolate ZIKV also in some populations of *Aedes albopictus* (tiger mosquito) coming from Gabon. As this mosquito has become very common even in the temperate climates of the northern hemisphere, such as in North America, the Italian peninsula, and other areas of the Mediterranean basin, it could in the future pose a serious risk for the expansion of the virus even in these areas of the planet. In this regard, however, there are no documented cases of transmission of the virus in Europe by this mosquito. Like the other viruses in this family, ZIKV is enveloped by an icosahedral capside and the genome consists of a single positive-sense RNA helix, 10,794 nucleotides long. From a phylogenetic point of view, it is closely related to the Spondweni Virus, a virus that forms a group of its own (clade) within the *Flavivirus* genus with ZIKV. It shares the same structural characteristics and replication cycle with the other members of the genre, as well as the genetic organization itself, except for the 3' untranslated region (UTR). Other members belonging to the same genus are the Ilheus Virus (ILHV), the virus that causes Rocio encephalitis or Rocio Virus (ROCV), and Saint-Louis Encephalitis Virus (SLEV). There are cases of possible viral co-infection such as dengue + chikungunya + zika. Zika fever is predominantly contracted by arthropod (mosquitoes) bites, although direct infection through blood products or by sexual means is possible, given the presence of virions in the semen of affected men. Main animal reservoirs of infection are primates, some large mammals (hippopotamuses, impalas, elephants, goats, sheep, hartebeests, lions, wildebeests, and zebras) and rodents. During the first week of infection, ZIKV is present in the bloodstream and can be isolated by the subject's blood. Many mosquito species have been identified as vectors of the virus, belonging to the genera *Aedes*, *Anopheles*, *Mansonia*, and *Eretmapodites*. In hot climates, the main vector is *A. africanus* and *A. aegypti* and, to a lesser extent, *A. polynesiensis*, *A. unilineatus*, *A. vittatus*, and *A. hensilli*. During the zika fever epidemic in Yap Island in 2007, *Aedes hensilli* was identified as the main vector. In the other more temperate climates, a potential vector could become the tiger mosquito (*Aedes albopictus*), abundantly distributed throughout the world. However, no cases of transmission of the virus in European areas have been documented although this mosquito is now quite common in some areas such as the Italian peninsula or other areas of the Mediterranean basin and central Europe.

The known transmission routes are: perinatal, sexual transmission, saliva, urine, semen, and breast milk. The possibility of maternal-fetal contagion is also likely, since the virus was found inside the placenta and in the amniotic fluid of pregnant patients, with consequent teratogenic effects reported on the embryo, especially in the first trimester of pregnancy. It is reported the possibility of virus transmission with the saliva/kiss, but this way is very remote, due to the low viral load in the saliva. The possibility of sperm transmission, on the contrary, is instead documented, having been officially confirmed in February 2016 the second case of transmission of the virus by sexual means, in Texas, in a woman infected by the partner returned from a trip to South America. A Brazilian study published by *The Lancet* on February 17th, 2016 suggested the possible confirmation of maternal-fetal transmission with amniotic fluid (vertical transmission). The strain affecting Brazil in 2016 is genetically related to that found in French Polynesia in 2013; in addition, researchers wrote that this strain is responsible for the cases of microcephaly found in Brazil to an abnormally high extent compared to before ZIKV epidemic, even though there is still no definitive evidence of the tropism of the virus on human nerve cells. The virus was isolated in 1947 from a specimen of mulatto macaque present in the Zika Forest of Uganda, and later in 1968 it was isolated for the first time in humans in Nigeria. From 1951 to 1981, similar human specimens were also positive in Uganda, Tanzania, Egypt, Central African Republic, Sierra Leone, Senegal, and Gabon. In Asia, it was found in India, Malaysia, Philippines, Thailand, Vietnam, and Indonesia where it was found in 2006. The first known zika outbreak from Africa occurred in 2007 in Yap Island, Micronesia. ZIKV was found in 2015 also in Colombia, Suriname, El Salvador, Guatemala, Cape Verde, Fiji, Vanuatu, Samoa, New Caledonia, Solomon Islands, Indonesia, Mexico, and Brazil. The World Health Organization (WHO) declared in February 2016 that ZIKV epidemic is a Public Health Emergency of International Concern (PHEIC) or "an international public health urgency"; just a few months before the start of the 2016 Olympics that would take place in Brazil in August. Still, the WHO, waiting for a vaccine to be prepared, suggests resorting to therapeutic abortion to the governments of the Countries involved in the epidemic, in order to avoid possible explosive growth of cases of microcephaly in the offspring of infected pregnant women. Studies that have analyzed the whole RNA of the infectious agent have demonstrated high genomic homology between the Latin-American stock and the one that circulated in the Pacific between 2013 and 2014. In 2015, in Brazil, the prevalence of new cases was estimated between 440,000 and 1,300,000, while native cases were recorded in Colombia, El Salvador, Guatemala, Mexico, Paraguay, Puerto Rico, and Venezuela. Furthermore, again in Brazil, in 2015 there were as many as 3,500 cases of microcephaly in infants, compared to the previous 150 cases/year. In healthy United States (US) travelers, returning from Countries where the virus is endemic, serological positivity to specific antibodies has been reported. These imported cases are destined to increase and may lead to the local spread of the virus in some areas of the US. *The New York Times* of January 17th, 2016 reported the first US case of microcephaly in a newborn, born in Ohau in Hawaii, whose mother had stayed in Brazil for several months during pregnancy. An additional case has been reported in Texas. On January 27th, 2016, the first case of zika in Argentina was confirmed. In Spain, the first case in Europe of pregnant woman infected by ZIKV was reported on February 4th, 2016. As of February 6th, 2016, 9 cases of ZIKV infection were reported in Italy. The first case of ZIKV disease in China was reported on February 9th, 2016.

It is hypothesized that the infection starts from dendritic cells close to the inoculum site, followed by development in the satellite lymph nodes and then through the bloodstream. Typically, Flaviviruses replicate in the cytoplasm, but ZIKV antigen has also been found in the nuclei of infected cells. The incubation period of the disease after the puncture with the vector is about 10 days. The disease caused by this virus is asymptomatic in 25% of cases (according to the Centers for Disease Control and Prevention [CDC], 80% of people infected with the virus are asymptomatic), or causes mild symptomatology, as in dengue, with which it can be confused. In this case, symptoms may be mild fever, rash (exanthema), conjunctivitis, and headache. ZIKV infection is usually mild, with symptoms lasting only a few days. Since there is no etiological therapy that reduces infection, treatment focuses essentially on alleviating symptoms and preventing further infection. Prevention and control are based on reducing the development of mosquitoes of the *Aedes* genus and minimizing the contact between vector mosquitoes and people, by means of barriers (repellents, mosquito nets), reducing water stagnations that support development mosquito pups and larvae, and breaking down, with disinfestation, the population of adult mosquitoes in communities at risk. The differential diagnosis should be made with the following infections: dengue, leptospirosis, malaria, rickettsiosis, group A streptococcus, rubella, measles, parvovirus, enterovirus, adenovirus, alphavirus (Chikungunya Virus [CHIKV], Mayaro Virus [MAYV], Ross River Virus [RRV], Barmah Forest Virus [BFV], O'Nyong-Nyong Virus [ONNV], and Sindbis Virus [SINV]). The diagnostic tests for ZIKV are: deoxy-ribonucleic acid (DNA) reverse transcription polymerase chain reaction (RT-PCR) on serum. Immunoglobulins M (IgM), neutralizing antibodies that develop, generally, towards the end of the first week of specific virus disease, are in cross-reaction with the related Flaviviruses (e.g., Dengue Virus [DENV] and Yellow Fever Virus [YFV]); the virus is common and can be difficult to distinguish. In order to refine the diagnosis, specific tests have been introduced to distinguish zika from other Flaviviruses. The mechanisms with which the clinical complications of zika infection are expressed seem to be due to a duplication/amplification of the centrosomes of the nerve cells. This causes in the mice neural delayed mitosis, increased apoptosis, with stem cell disorientation, premature neuronal differentiation, and reduction of the number of progenitor cells, all mechanisms that well explain microcephaly cases. Infection with this virus in pregnant women is believed to result in microcephaly and fetal malformations in the baby. In 2015, in the North of Brazil there was a very important increase in cases of microcephaly, whose cause seems to be closely related to ZIKV infection in pregnant women, even asymptomatic. The CDC in Atlanta, US, in January 2016 issued level two alert for pregnant or at risk to be pregnant women so that, if possible, they avoid going to Countries at risk (Brazil, Colombia, El Salvador, French Guiana, Guatemala, Haiti, Honduras, Martinique, Mexico, Panama, Paraguay, Puerto Rico, Dominican Republic, Suriname, and Venezuela) or observe adequate precautions. On autopsy examination of a 29-week fetus, aborted by a woman with zika fever in the first trimester of pregnancy, it was observed that she presented: "almost complete agyria (lack of brain convolutions), hydrocephalus, and multifocal dystrophic calcifications in the cortex and subcortical white matter, with associated cortical displacement and mild focal inflammation." ZIKV was found in fetal brain tissue and it was possible to study and have its complete genome. With this work, the relationship between ZIKV and microcephaly in pregnancy was confirmed. There is a correlation between ZIKV infection and Guillain-Barré syndrome (GBS): 74 cases of this disease were diagnosed in individuals already affected by the infection in French Polynesia. On February 6th, 2016, three deaths were confirmed due to this severe syndrome in subjects with previous ZIKV infection. Research has shown that 2.4 patients every 10,000 affected by ZIKV get GBS after a few days of infection, with a frequency about 20 times greater than expected cases; of these, 3-5% undergo mortal complications. This causes serious concern for the health systems and populations of Countries affected by the zika outbreak. A report from the European CDC (ECDC) indicates that in addition to an increase in the number of cases of GBS, there may also be a significant increase in cases of encephalitis, meningoencephalitis, facial paralysis, and myelitis. In February 2016, a Brazilian case-report correlated hypertensive uveitis with zika infection. Other Brazilian researchers have found important malformations of the optic nerve and of the macula in neonates affected by post-zika microcephaly.

Since no specific antiviral treatment exists, therapy is essentially based on rest, fluids, and the use of antipyretics if needed. Because of the symptomatic similarity, and up to the precise identification of the infectious agent, it is advisable to consider patients with suspected zika in the same way as suspected dengue or chikungunya. For this reason, the intake of aspirin or other non-steroidal anti-inflammatory drugs (NSAID) may be inadvisable to reduce the risk of bleeding, as in dengue. The Authorities believe that this virus can have some impact also in transfusion medicine. In fact, the ECDC requires 28-day postponement of blood donation in subjects who have had possible symptoms of the disease, and 14-day one in those who returned from Countries at risk. All zika patients, or suspected ones, must also be immediately adequately isolated from the possible contact with mosquitoes, in order to reduce the risk of local transmission. First, avoid, where possible, travel in the epidemic areas, above all for pregnant women or women at risk of pregnancy during stay abroad. Aggressive methods of prevention against vectors (mosquitoes), including repellents based on N,N-diethyl-meta-toluamide (DEET), picaridin, and Insect Repellent 3535 (IR3535) are advisable; these are considered safe even during pregnancy. Serological tests, including RT-PCR, should be made on women who have returned from stays in areas endemic to zika fever.

Chapter 2 - Multiple myeloma is characterized by the expansion of monoclonal plasma cells in the bone marrow. In about 95% of cases the aberrant plasma cells produce a monoclonal immunoglobulin called monoclonal component that can be considered a marker of the disease. Multiple myeloma diagnostic criteria include: bone marrow plasmacytosis, the presence of monoclonal protein in the serum and/or urine and the presence of one of these signs and symptoms, the so-called CRAB manifestation: hypercalcemia (C), renal insufficiency (R), bone marrow insufficiency (especially anemia) (A) and/or osteolytic lesions (B). The more recent revision of these criteria allows the diagnosis of multiple myeloma even in absence of the CRAB manifestation, if one of these condition is present: >60% of plasma cells in the bone marrow, a value of serum Free Light Chains ratio>100, or>1 focal lesion identified by magnetic resonance.

Over the last few decades, the introduction of intensive treatments, such as high dose chemotherapy followed by autologous stem cell transplantation and novel agents, including immunomodulatory drugs (thalidomide, lenalidomide and pomalidomide), proteosome inhibitors (bortezomib, carfilzomib, ixazomib), and monoclonal antibodies (elotuzumab and daratumumab), has markedly improved the outcome of multiple myeloma patients. Three-drugs combinations, including at least bortezomib or lenalidomide, are now routinely used as induction therapy for young newly diagnosed patients, followed by high-dose chemotherapy and autologous transplantation. Bortezomib and lenalidomide are also commonly used as induction therapy for elderly patients within different regimens.

Treatment for relapse/refractory patients includes combinations of new-generation agents (such as carfilzomib, ixazomib, elotuzumab and daratumumab with lenalidomide and dexamethasone or daratumumab with bortezomib and dexamethasone) but also monotherapy (pomalidomide or daratumumab).

A deep knowledge of the toxicities of all these novel drugs is mandatory to better manage all potential side effects and to reduce the risk of treatment discontinuation or serious adverse events.

Given the wide range of therapeutic regimens that are now available, the choice of the best treatment cannot be so obvious. Therefore, it must be necessary to draw homogeneous therapeutic guidelines to identify the best sequence of treatment to adopt during the course of the disease and also the precise timing (at biochemical relapse or clinical relapse).

Moreover, a deeper characterization of patients (by phenotype, cytogenetic and molecular biology) and the evaluation of minimal residual disease would guide the choice in the treatment of multiple myeloma patients.

Chapter 3 - Sudden sensorineural hearing loss (SSNHL) is a common clinical entity and defined as a rapid onset of hearing impairment, occurring within three days. It has an audiometric criteria identified as a decrease in hearing of at least 30 dB over three contiguous test frequencies in one or both ears. It has a significant effect on quality of life. As the 88% of SSNHL cases is idiopathic at presentation, there is usually no known exact specific etiologic factor. However, multiple reasons such as vascular compromise and associated cochlear ischemia or viral etiologies, etc. have been presumed and the treatment modalities have been empiric. Although oral steroid therapy is the mainstay treatment in clinical practice, in most of the centers, several different treatment modalities proposed in the literature. Hyperbaric oxygen therapy (HBOT), which has been used for SSNHL treatment since 1979, exposes a patient to 100% oxygen at a pressure level higher than 1 atmosphere absolute in a specially designed sealed chamber. This facilitates a delivery of increased partial pressure of oxygen to the tissues. Based on this fact, it is thought that HBOT may prevent damage caused from ischemia by improving the supply of oxygen to the inner ear and result in an improvement in hearing. This review focuses on the benefits and harms of HBOT in treating SSNHL.

Chapter 4 - *Introduction:* Since its advent, ruxolitinib has been shown to be a very effective treatment for myelofibrosis and polycythemia vera. Drugs can sometimes have uses beyond the official approved indication.

Hypereosinophilic syndrome (HES) is a hematologic disorder in which the eosinophils overproliferate. JAK inhibitors have also demonstrated efficacy in treating HES, as well as in the treatments of alopecia and madarosis.

Method: Review of literature

Conclusion: Ruxolitinib has beneficial effects in treating other conditions, considered off-label. These include HES, alopecia areata, and madarosis. Physicians and patients should be aware of the side effects of these JAK inhibitors. Further investigation is needed to ascertain whether ruxolitinib or other interleukin inhibitors can aid in the treatment of additional conditions.

Chapter 5 - Despite significant advances, the adverse health effects of benzene exposure in children have rarely been studied. Children at various developmental stages have unique physical risk factors when exposed to toxic chemicals such as benzene due to their levels of mobility, oxygen consumption, hormonal production, and overall growth. They are more susceptible to leukemogenesis because their hematopoietic cell populations are differentiating and undergoing maturation. The susceptibility to benzene may vary due to its effect that arises, in part, from genetic variations in its metabolism, DNA repair, genomic stability, and immune function. The pharmacokinetics of benzene differ widely between children and adults due to childrens' incomplete metabolic systems, rapid tissue regeneration, immature host defenses, activity patterns, and high rates of infection by respiratory pathogens. Thus, exposure to benzene can cause deleterious health effects among children. Given the importance of the toxicity of benzene, this chapter provides summaries of the current scientific knowledge and understanding of the clinical findings and health consequences of benzene exposure among children.

Chapter 6 - Benzene, a monocyclic aromatic hydrocarbon, is a carcinogenic liquid. Before the 1920s, benzene was frequently used as an industrial solvent, particularly for degreasing metals. When its toxicity becomes obvious, it is replaced by other solvents for applications requiring direct exposure of the user. Benzene is used for the most part as an intermediate in the synthesis of other chemical compounds. A hybrid

[Genetic algorithm (GA/Artificial neural network (ANN)] QSAR model was developed for the prediction of aqueous toxicity. The data concerning 92 substituted benzenes was separated into two disjoined subsets, respectively 74 elements for calculating and testing of the model, and 18 elements for its external validation. Theoretical molecular descriptors were calculated by using commercially available software of molecular modeling. The size of the model was determined by optimizing the FIT of KUBINYI, and the selection of the descriptors realized by genetic algorithm. The values of the statistical parameters (R^2, Q^2, Q^2ext, SDEC, SDEP, SDEPext) obtained attest relevance of the developed model.

In: Advances in Health and Disease
Editor: Lowell T. Duncan
ISBN: 978-1-53616-380-3

Chapter 1

ZIKA VIRUS INFECTION: A NEW THREAD FOR PREGNANCY

***Ciro Comparetto*[1,*] *and Franco Borruto*[2]**
[1]Obstetrician and Gynecologist, Florence, Italy
[2]Consultant in Health Policy of the Government of Monaco, Principality of Monaco

ABSTRACT

Zika Virus (ZIKV) is a ribonucleic acid (RNA) virus of the *Flaviviridae* family, genus *Flavivirus*, *Spondweni* group, *Zika* species, isolated for the first time in 1947 from a primate in Uganda, in the Zika Forest, a natural reserve near Entebbe. In the years 2010, there were occurrences of the disease in all continents and isolated cases were also recorded in Europe, on subjects who were returning from travel in tropical areas and without any form of transmission of the virus in Europe. In humans, it causes a disease known as "zika" or zika fever. The virus is closely related to those that cause dengue, yellow fever, West Nile encephalitis, and Japanese encephalitis, all transmitted mainly by insect bites and therefore called "arthropode-borne viruses" (arboviruses).

* Corresponding Author's Email: cicomp@tin.it.

The virus is transmitted by numerous mosquitoes of the genus *Aedes*, in equatorial environments especially by *Aedes aegypti*. Studies on the vectors involved in the transmission of the virus have allowed to isolate ZIKV also in some populations of *Aedes albopictus* (tiger mosquito) coming from Gabon. As this mosquito has become very common even in the temperate climates of the northern hemisphere, such as in North America, the Italian peninsula, and other areas of the Mediterranean basin, it could in the future pose a serious risk for the expansion of the virus even in these areas of the planet. In this regard, however, there are no documented cases of transmission of the virus in Europe by this mosquito. Like the other viruses in this family, ZIKV is enveloped by an icosahedral capside and the genome consists of a single positive-sense RNA helix, 10,794 nucleotides long. From a phylogenetic point of view, it is closely related to the Spondweni Virus, a virus that forms a group of its own (clade) within the *Flavivirus* genus with ZIKV. It shares the same structural characteristics and replication cycle with the other members of the genre, as well as the genetic organization itself, except for the 3' untranslated region (UTR). Other members belonging to the same genus are the Ilheus Virus (ILHV), the virus that causes Rocio encephalitis or Rocio Virus (ROCV), and Saint-Louis Encephalitis Virus (SLEV). There are cases of possible viral co-infection such as dengue + chikungunya + zika. Zika fever is predominantly contracted by arthropod (mosquitoes) bites, although direct infection through blood products or by sexual means is possible, given the presence of virions in the semen of affected men. Main animal reservoirs of infection are primates, some large mammals (hippopotamuses, impalas, elephants, goats, sheep, hartebeests, lions, wildebeests, and zebras) and rodents. During the first week of infection, ZIKV is present in the bloodstream and can be isolated by the subject's blood. Many mosquito species have been identified as vectors of the virus, belonging to the genera *Aedes*, *Anopheles*, *Mansonia*, and *Eretmapodites*. In hot climates, the main vector is *A. africanus* and *A. aegypti* and, to a lesser extent, *A. polynesiensis*, *A. unilineatus*, *A. vittatus*, and *A. hensilli*. During the zika fever epidemic in Yap Island in 2007, *Aedes hensilli* was identified as the main vector. In the other more temperate climates, a potential vector could become the tiger mosquito (*Aedes albopictus*), abundantly distributed throughout the world. However, no cases of transmission of the virus in European areas have been documented although this mosquito is now quite common in some areas such as the Italian peninsula or other areas of the Mediterranean basin and central Europe.

The known transmission routes are: perinatal, sexual transmission, saliva, urine, semen, and breast milk. The possibility of maternal-fetal contagion is also likely, since the virus was found inside the placenta and in the amniotic fluid of pregnant patients, with consequent teratogenic effects reported on the embryo, especially in the first trimester of pregnancy. It is reported the possibility of virus transmission with the saliva/kiss, but this way is very remote, due to the low viral load in the saliva. The possibility of sperm transmission, on the contrary, is instead documented, having been officially confirmed in February 2016 the second case of transmission of the virus by sexual means, in Texas, in a woman infected by the partner returned from a trip to South America. A Brazilian study published by *The Lancet* on February 17th, 2016 suggested the possible confirmation of maternal-fetal transmission with amniotic fluid (vertical transmission). The strain affecting Brazil in 2016 is genetically related to that found in French Polynesia in 2013; in addition, researchers wrote that this strain is responsible for the cases of microcephaly found in Brazil to an abnormally high extent compared to before ZIKV epidemic, even though there is still no definitive evidence of the tropism of the virus on human nerve cells. The virus was isolated in 1947 from a specimen of mulatto macaque present in the Zika Forest of Uganda, and later in 1968 it was isolated for the first time in humans in Nigeria. From 1951 to 1981, similar human specimens were also positive in Uganda, Tanzania, Egypt, Central African Republic, Sierra Leone, Senegal, and Gabon. In Asia, it was found in India, Malaysia, Philippines, Thailand, Vietnam, and Indonesia where it was found in 2006. The first known zika outbreak from Africa occurred in 2007 in Yap Island, Micronesia. ZIKV was found in 2015 also in Colombia, Suriname, El Salvador, Guatemala, Cape Verde, Fiji, Vanuatu, Samoa, New Caledonia, Solomon Islands, Indonesia, Mexico, and Brazil. The World Health Organization (WHO) declared in February 2016 that ZIKV epidemic is a Public Health Emergency of International Concern (PHEIC) or "an international public health urgency"; just a few months before the start of the 2016 Olympics that would take place in Brazil in August. Still, the WHO, waiting for a vaccine to be prepared, suggests resorting to therapeutic abortion to the governments of the Countries involved in the epidemic, in order to avoid possible explosive growth of cases of microcephaly in the offspring of infected pregnant women. Studies that have analyzed the whole RNA of the infectious agent have demonstrated high genomic homology between the Latin-American stock and the one that circulated in the Pacific between 2013 and 2014. In 2015, in Brazil, the prevalence of new cases was estimated between 440,000 and 1,300,000, while native cases were recorded in Colombia, El Salvador, Guatemala, Mexico, Paraguay, Puerto Rico, and Venezuela. Furthermore, again in Brazil, in 2015 there were as many as 3,500 cases of microcephaly in infants, compared to the previous 150 cases/year. In healthy United States (US) travelers, returning from Countries where the virus is endemic, serological positivity to specific antibodies has been reported. These imported cases are destined to increase and may lead to the local spread of the virus in some areas of the US. *The New York Times* of January 17th, 2016 reported the first US case of microcephaly in a newborn, born in Ohau in Hawaii, whose mother had stayed in Brazil for several months during pregnancy. An additional case has been reported in Texas. On January 27th, 2016, the first case of zika in Argentina was confirmed. In Spain, the first case in Europe of pregnant woman infected by ZIKV was reported on February 4th, 2016. As of February 6th, 2016, 9 cases of ZIKV infection were reported in Italy. The first case of ZIKV disease in China was reported on February 9th, 2016.

It is hypothesized that the infection starts from dendritic cells close to the inoculum site, followed by development in the satellite lymph nodes and then through the bloodstream. Typically, Flaviviruses replicate in the cytoplasm, but ZIKV antigen has also been found in the nuclei of infected cells. The incubation period of the disease after the puncture with the vector is about 10 days. The disease caused by this virus is asymptomatic in 25% of cases (according to the Centers for Disease Control and Prevention [CDC], 80% of people infected with the virus are asymptomatic), or causes mild symptomatology, as in dengue, with which it can be confused. In this case, symptoms may be mild fever, rash (exanthema), conjunctivitis, and headache. ZIKV infection is usually mild, with symptoms lasting only a few days. Since there is no etiological therapy that reduces infection, treatment focuses essentially on alleviating symptoms and preventing further infection. Prevention and control are based on reducing the development of mosquitoes of the *Aedes* genus and minimizing the contact between vector mosquitoes and people, by means of barriers (repellents, mosquito nets), reducing water stagnations that support development mosquito pups and larvae, and breaking down, with disinfestation, the population of adult mosquitoes in communities at risk. The differential diagnosis should be made with the following infections: dengue, leptospirosis, malaria, rickettsiosis, group A streptococcus, rubella, measles, parvovirus, enterovirus, adenovirus, alphavirus (Chikungunya Virus [CHIKV], Mayaro Virus [MAYV], Ross River Virus [RRV], Barmah Forest Virus [BFV], O'Nyong-Nyong Virus [ONNV], and Sindbis Virus [SINV]). The diagnostic tests for ZIKV are: deoxy-ribonucleic acid (DNA) reverse transcription polymerase chain reaction (RT-PCR) on serum. Immunoglobulins M (IgM), neutralizing antibodies that develop, generally, towards the end of the first week of specific virus disease, are in cross-reaction with the related Flaviviruses (e.g., Dengue Virus [DENV] and Yellow Fever Virus [YFV]); the virus is common and can be difficult to distinguish. In order to refine the diagnosis, specific tests have been introduced to distinguish zika from other Flaviviruses. The mechanisms with which the clinical complications of zika infection are expressed seem to be due to a duplication/amplification of the centrosomes of the nerve cells. This causes in the mice neural delayed mitosis, increased apoptosis, with stem cell disorientation, premature neuronal differentiation, and reduction of the number of progenitor cells, all mechanisms that well explain microcephaly cases. Infection with this virus in pregnant women is believed to result in microcephaly and fetal malformations in the baby. In 2015, in the North of Brazil there was a very important increase in cases of microcephaly, whose cause seems to be closely related to ZIKV infection in pregnant women, even asymptomatic. The CDC in Atlanta, US, in January 2016 issued level two alert for pregnant or at risk to be pregnant women so that, if possible, they avoid going to Countries at risk (Brazil, Colombia, El Salvador, French Guiana, Guatemala, Haiti, Honduras, Martinique, Mexico, Panama, Paraguay, Puerto Rico, Dominican Republic, Suriname, and Venezuela) or observe adequate precautions. On autopsy examination of a 29-week fetus, aborted by a woman with zika fever in the first trimester of pregnancy, it was observed that she presented: "almost complete agyria (lack of brain convolutions), hydrocephalus, and multifocal dystrophic calcifications in the cortex and subcortical white matter, with associated cortical displacement and mild focal inflammation." ZIKV was found in fetal brain tissue and it was possible to study and have its complete genome. With this work, the relationship between ZIKV and microcephaly in pregnancy was confirmed. There is a correlation between ZIKV infection and Guillain-Barré syndrome (GBS): 74 cases of this disease were diagnosed in individuals already affected by the infection in French Polynesia. On February 6th, 2016, three deaths were confirmed due to this severe syndrome in subjects with previous ZIKV infection. Research has shown that 2.4 patients every 10,000 affected by ZIKV get GBS after a few days of infection, with a frequency about 20 times greater than expected cases; of these, 3-5% undergo mortal complications. This causes serious concern for the health systems and populations of Countries affected by the zika outbreak. A report from the European CDC (ECDC) indicates that in addition to an increase in the number of cases of GBS, there may also be a significant increase in cases of encephalitis, meningoencephalitis, facial paralysis, and myelitis. In February 2016, a Brazilian case-report correlated hypertensive uveitis with zika infection. Other Brazilian researchers have found important malformations of the optic nerve and of the macula in neonates affected by post-zika microcephaly.

Since no specific antiviral treatment exists, therapy is essentially based on rest, fluids, and the use of antipyretics if needed. Because of the symptomatic similarity, and up to the precise identification of the infectious agent, it is advisable to consider patients with suspected zika in the same way as suspected dengue or chikungunya. For this reason, the intake of aspirin or other non-steroidal anti-inflammatory drugs (NSAID) may be inadvisable to reduce the risk of bleeding, as in dengue. The Authorities believe that this virus can have some impact also in transfusion medicine. In fact, the ECDC requires 28-day postponement of blood donation in subjects who have had possible symptoms of the disease, and 14-day one in those who returned from Countries at risk. All zika patients, or suspected ones, must also be immediately adequately isolated from the possible contact with mosquitoes, in order to reduce the risk of local transmission. First, avoid, where possible, travel in the epidemic areas, above all for pregnant women or women at risk of pregnancy during stay abroad. Aggressive methods of prevention against vectors (mosquitoes), including repellents based on N,N-diethyl-meta-toluamide (DEET), picaridin, and Insect Repellent 3535 (IR3535) are advisable; these are considered safe even during pregnancy. Serological tests, including RT-PCR, should be made on women who have returned from stays in areas endemic to zika fever.

Keywords: Zyka Virus, pregnancy, microcephaly, Guillain-Barré syndrome

INTRODUCTION

At present, one of greatest concerns of medical caregivers is the arthropod-borne virus (arbovirus) Zika Virus (ZIKV). ZIKV is a mosquito-borne single-stranded ribonucleic acid (RNA) virus, member of *Flaviviridae* family in the genus *Flavivirus*, closely related to Japanese Encephalitis Virus (JEV), West Nile Virus (WNV), Dengue Virus (DENV), Chikungunya Virus (CHIKV), and Yellow Fever Virus (YFV). ZIKV spread across Africa and Asia to the Americas, in part owing to unique genomic evolutionary conditions and pressures resulting in specific human disease manifestations, complications, and pathogenesis. The virus is transmitted primarily through the bite of infected blood-sucking *Aedes aegypti* and *Aedes albopictus* (*Stegomyia*) mosquitoes, but other routes of transmission include sexual, mother-to-fetus during pregnancy, mother-to-infant at delivery, laboratory exposure, and, possibly, transfusion of blood products. Historically, ZIKV infection was considered a sporadic, relatively mild disease. Although ZIKV infection generally causes only mild symptoms in some infected individuals, it is associated with a range of neuro-immunological disorders, including meningoencephalitis and myelitis, due to a reduction of proliferative zones and disrupted cortical layers and synaptogenesis. An increased incidence of Guillain-Barré syndrome (GBS), an immune-mediated neuropathy of the peripheral nervous system (PNS), has also been reported in ZIKV-infected patients. Moreover, the amniotic fluids, blood cord, and miscarriage tissues of mothers have been detected with ZIKV, which indicates that the virus either gets transferred from mother to fetus or seeks direct entry in the fetus, causing microcephaly and other brain anomalies in the newborn babies and even abortion [1]. Reports have highlighted the sexual transmission of ZIKV, as it has been detected in the semen and saliva of affected persons [2]. With the increased number of cases, new complications such as ocular involvement and severe thrombocytopenia have been reported. Head and neck manifestations include conjunctivitis, retro-orbital pain, cephalgia, and odynophagia [3, 4].

Though ZIKV has been reported for quite a long time, its rapid emergence, new modes of transmission, and, more importantly, the congenital anomalies associated with it have made the situation worse. Since its first discovery in the Zika Forest in Uganda in 1947, incidentally isolated from a sentinel Rhesus monkey and from mosquitoes in the same forest the following year, and its first human infection in 1952, ZIKV has continued to expand its geographic range, from equatorial Africa and Asia to the Pacific Islands, then further afield to South and Central America and the Caribbean. Although entomological and virologic surveillance have reported ZIKV enzootic activity in diverse Countries of Africa and Asia, few human cases were reported until 2007, when a zika fever epidemic took place in Micronesia. The rapid expansion of ZIKV in the South and Central America has recently gained medical attention, emphasizing the capacity of ZIKV to spread to non-endemic regions. In the context of West Africa, the World Health Organization (WHO) Collaborating Center for Arboviruses and Hemorrhagic Fever at Institute Pasteur of Dakar reported the periodic circulation of ZIKV since 1968. Currently, ZIKV is actively circulating not only in much of Latin America and its neighbors but also in parts of the Pacific Islands and Southeast Asia. Since local mosquito-borne transmission of ZIKV was first reported in Brazil in early 2015, the virus has spread rapidly to several surrounding Countries, with active transmission reported in at least 61 Countries and territories worldwide, including the United States (US) and there is concern about the spread of the virus in areas where competent vectors are present. Though it is asymptomatic in maximum number of cases, the serious complications of the infection should be prevented at the earliest. Despite its emergence as an important public health problem, however, little is known about ZIKV biology, and neither vaccine nor effective therapies currently exist for treating patients infected with ZIKV, thus treatment is supportive and prevention is based on individual measures and on vectors control. But research continues and hopefully, success is not far off. The right information about this infection should reach patients as well as physicians. It will prevent unnecessary panic [5, 6]. A large number of studies have been published in the last five years, revealing the structure of the virus, how it is transmitted, and how it affects human cells. Many different animal models have been developed, which recapitulate several features of ZIKV disease and its neurological consequences. Moreover, several vaccine candidates are now in active pre-clinical development, and three of them have already entered phase I clinical trials. Likewise, many different compounds targeting viral and cellular components are being tested in in vitro and in experimental animal models [7, 8].

ZIKV has emerged as a global public health threat over the last decade, with the accelerated geographic spread of the virus noted during the last 10 years. The WHO predicted that millions of cases of ZIKV were likely to occur in the Americas during the last five years. These projections, in conjunction with suspected ZIKV-associated increase in newborn microcephaly cases, resulted in activation of the Center for Disease Control and Prevention (CDC)'s Emergency Operations Center (EOC) on January 22nd, 2016, to ensure a coordinated response and timely dissemination of information, and led the WHO to declare a Public Health Emergency of International Concern (PHEIC) on February 1st, 2016. ZIKV-associated illness is characterized by an incubation period of three to 12 days. Most patients (i.e., ~80%) remain asymptomatic after contracting the virus. When symptomatic, clinical presentation is usually mild and consists of a self-limiting febrile illness that lasts approximately two to seven days. Among common clinical manifestations are fever, arthralgia, non-purulent conjunctivitis, myalgia, headache, maculopapular rash, and weakness. Hospitalization and complication rates are low, with fatalities being extremely rare. Newborn microcephaly, the most devastating and insidious complication associated with ZIKV, has been described in the offspring of women who became infected while pregnant. Much remains to be elucidated about the timing of ZIKV infection in the context of the temporal progression of pregnancy, the corresponding *in utero* fetal development stages, and the risk of microcephaly. Without further knowledge of the pathophysiology involved, the true risk of ZIKV to the unborn remains difficult to quantify. Accurate, portable, and inexpensive point-of-care testing is required to better identify cases and manage the current and future outbreaks of ZIKV, including optimization of preventive approaches and the identification of more effective risk-reduction strategies. ZIKV testing is recommended for persons with possible exposure (those who have traveled to or live in an area with active transmission, or persons who had sex without a condom with a person with possible exposure) if they have symptoms consistent with ZIKV disease. Testing is also recommended for pregnant women with possible exposure, regardless of whether symptoms are present. Clinicians should understand the infection, its diagnosis, and testing, and monitor pregnant women for travel history to outbreak regions and for the presence of clinical symptoms. Patient education on preventive measures offers the best option to avoid ZIKV infection. Given the rapid geographic spread of ZIKV in recent years, a coordinated local, regional, and global effort is needed to generate sufficient resources and political traction to effectively halt and contain further expansion of the current outbreak [9, 10]. During the past years, public health agencies and researchers worldwide have collaborated to protect pregnant women, inform clinicians and the public, and advance knowledge about ZIKV. The primary methods of prevention include avoiding bites of infected *Aedes* mosquitoes and reducing the risk of sexual transmission. To protect pregnant women and their fetuses and infants from the effects of ZIKV infection during pregnancy, public health activities must focus on preventing mosquito-borne transmission through vector control and personal protective practices, preventing sexual transmission by advising abstention from sex or consistent and correct use of condoms, and preventing unintended pregnancies by reducing barriers to access to highly effective reversible contraception [11]. Pregnant women should not travel to areas with active ZIKV transmission, and men and women who are planning to conceive in the near future should consider avoiding non-essential travel to these areas [12-15].

MICROBIOLOGY

Many members of the genus *Flavivirus* are the agents of important diseases of humans, livestock, and wildlife. Until the last 10 years, no complete genome sequence was available for the three African viruses, Bagaza Virus (BAGV), Kedougou Virus (KEDV), and ZIKV, each representing a distinct virus subgroup according to the latest virus classification. It has been obtained a complete genome sequence of each of those three viruses and characterized the open reading frames (ORF) with respect to gene sizes, cleavage sites, potential glycosylation sites, distribution of cysteine residues, and unique motifs [16]. Whereas much is known about the biology of related Flaviviruses, the unique features of ZIKV pathogenesis, including infection of the fetus, persistence in immune-privileged sites, and sexual transmission, have presented new challenges. The rapid development of cell culture and animal models has facilitated a new appreciation of ZIKV biology. This knowledge has created opportunities for the development of countermeasures, including multiple ZIKV vaccine candidates, which are advancing through clinical trials [17]. There are three genetic lineages of ZIKV: the East African, West African, and Asian lineages. Despite several reports on ZIKV, the genetic relationships among viral strains from West Africa remain poorly understood. ZIKV has possibly undergone recombination in nature and a loss of the N-linked glycosylation site (N154) in the envelope protein was a possible adaptive response to the *Aedes dalzieli* vector [18]. Despite the relatively short time interval, an intensive effort by the global scientific community has resulted in development of animal models to study multiple aspects of ZIKV biology. Several animal models have been established to investigate pathogenesis of ZIKV in adults, pregnant mothers, and developing fetuses [19, 20].

A mosquito-borne virus resulting in congenital anomalies is unique, and zika's ability to cause neurological defects on a large scale was a grim reminder of the Rubella Virus (RuV) epidemic in the 1950s. Over the past six years, studies have provided insight on how ZIKV infects cells and causes disease, but much remains unknown about the long-term risks of zika exposure on infant growth and development. The impact of ZIKV on pregnancy extends beyond microcephaly and may only first be identified in infancy. The virus has a long latency in semen and can be transmitted sexually. Transplacental passage occurs through infection of primary human placental macrophages, commonly referred to as Hofbauer cells, in the trophoblast. This has led to questions of how a Flavivirus is capable of crossing the placental barrier to reach the fetal brain. Permissive ZIKV infection of Hofbauer cells and placental villous fibroblasts has been demonstrated. It has been also demonstrated ZIKV infection of Hofbauer cells within the context of the tissue ex vivo using term placental villous explants. In addition to amplifying infectious virus within a usually inaccessible area, the putative migratory activities of Hofbauer cells may aid in dissemination of ZIKV to the fetal brain [21]. Hofbauer cells are placental villous macrophages of fetal origin that are present throughout pregnancy. Although Hofbauer cell populations are antigenically and morphologically heterogeneous, their epigenetic, antigenic, and functional profiles most closely resemble alternatively activated macrophages or what are referred to as M2a, M2b, M2c, and M2d polarity subtypes. Consistent with an M2-like profile, these cells play an important role in placental development including vasculo-genesis and angiogenesis. During placental inflammation, Hofbauer cells may produce pro-inflammatory cytokines or mediators that damage the villous cell barrier, and induce fibrotic responses within the villi as a continuum of chronic inflammation. However, to date, there is no evidence that Hofbauer cells become classically activated or adopt an M1 polarity phenotype that is able to kill microbes. To the contrary, their predominant M2-like qualities may be why these cells are ineffective in controlling most "TORCH" (*Toxoplasma gondii*, other, RuV, Cytomegalovirus [CMV], and Herpes Simplex Virus [HSV]) infections. Moreover, Hofbauer cells may contribute to vertical transmission of various pathogens to the fetus since they can harbor live virus and serve as reservoirs within the placenta [22]. Yet, placentas from fetuses with congenital ZIKV infection are concordant in not having viral-induced placental inflammation. Special stains reveal proliferation and prominent hyperplasia of Hofbauer cells in the chorionic villi of infected placentas. ZIKV infection is present in Hofbauer cells from second and third trimester placentas. Experimental studies and placentae from infected fetuses reveal that the spectrum of placental cell types infected with ZIKV is broader during the first trimester than later in gestation. Inflammatory abnormalities of the placenta are not a component of vertical transmission of ZIKV. The major placental response in second and third trimester transplacental ZIKV infection is proliferation and hyperplasia of Hofbauer cells, which also demonstrate viral infection [23].

Nevertheless, it is uncertain when during pregnancy the human conceptus is most vulnerable to the virus. The cells from term placentas, which resist infection, do not express genes encoding most attachment factors implicated in ZIKV entry but do express many genes associated with antiviral defense. By contrast, the embryonic stem cells (ESC)-derived trophoblasts possess a wide range of attachment factors for ZIKV entry and lack components of a robust antiviral response system. These cells, particularly areas of syncytiotrophoblast within the colonies, quickly become infected, produce infectious virus and undergo lysis within 48 h after exposure to low titers (multiplicity of infection >0.07) of an African lineage strain (MR766 Uganda [ZIKVU]) considered to be benign with regards to effects on fetal development. These data suggest that the developing fetus might be most vulnerable to ZIKV early in the first trimester before a protective zone of mature villous trophoblast has been established. Additionally, ZIKVU is highly trophic toward primitive trophoblast, which may put the early conceptus of an infected mother at high risk for destruction [24]. However, the cellular tropism and the mechanisms of ZIKV transmission to the fetus during early pregnancy are still largely unknown. ZIKV infects and damages tissue architecture of the maternal decidua basalis, the fetal placenta, and umbilical cord. ZIKV replicates differentially in a wide range of maternal and fetal cells, including decidual fibroblasts and macrophages, trophoblasts, Hofbauer cells, as well as umbilical cord mesenchymal stem cells (MSC). The striking cellular tropism of ZIKV and its cytopathic-induced tissue injury during the first trimester of pregnancy could provide an explanation for the irreversible congenital damages [25].

Secretory autophagy or exosome pathways may participate in this virus transfer. Autophagy modulators regulate autophagosome formation or membrane fusion with lysosomal vesicles and therefore inhibit viral nucleocapsid releasing or virus transfer to the fetus hypothetically. However, some autophagy modulators may enhance virus replication. Autophagy inhibitors may arrest placental development, while exaggeration of autophagy in human placenta may be associated with fetal intrauterine growth restriction (IUGR). Therefore, autophagy modulators should be used carefully due to their complex clinical effects. Alternatively, exosome-specific inhibitors might be also considered, although their safety of both maternal and fetal conditions must be carefully assessed before any advancement to human clinical trials [26]. A recent study investigated the key aspects of the ZIKV infectious life cycle. It has been demonstrated how inflammatory-activated stimulator of interferon (IFN) genes (STING)-dependent antiviral macroautophagy/autophagy is sufficient to restrict ZIKV infection in the *Drosophila melanogaster* brain. Additionally, this study provides further evidence for the ancestral function of autophagy in protecting host cells from viral invaders [27]. Circumstantial evidence has been presented in support of the hypothesis that ZIKV effects are due to an endogenous form of hypervitaminosis A resulting from ZIKV infection-induced damage to the liver and the spillage of stored vitamin A compounds ("retinoids") into the maternal and fetal circulation in toxic concentrations. Retinoids are mainly stored in the liver (about 80%) and are essential for numerous biological functions. In higher concentrations, retinoids are potentially cytotoxic, prooxidant, mutagenic, and teratogenic, especially if sudden shifts occur in their bodily distribution. Although liver involvement has not been mentioned specifically in recent reports, conventional liver enzyme testing underestimates the true extent of liver dysfunction. The proposed model could be tested by comparing retinoid concentration and expression profiles in microcephalic newborns of ZIKV-infected mothers and non-microcephalic newborn controls, and by correlating these profiles with measures of clinical severity [28].

Emerging evidence, mainly from *in vitro* studies, suggests that ZIKV may have direct effects on neuronal cells [29, 30]. ZIKV preferentially infects human neural progenitor cells (hNPC) and triggers cell apoptosis. ZIKV RNA has been identified in fetal brain tissue and brains of microcephalic infants who died and cerebrospinal fluid (CSF) and meninges of newborns. The increase in the number of GBS cases during the ZIKV outbreak in the Americas provides epidemiological evidence for the link between ZIKV infection and GBS. Less frequently reported ZIKV neurological complications include encephalitis/meningoencephalitis, acute disseminated encephalomyelitis, myelitis, cerebrovascular complications (ischemic infarction and vasculopathy), seizures and encephalopathy, sensory polyneuropathy, and sensory neuronopathy. Analysis of GBS incidence could serve as an epidemiological "marker" or sentinel for ZIKV disease and other neurological complications associated to ZIKV. An expanding spectrum of neurological complications associated with ZIKV infection is being recognized [31]. Recently, it has been demonstrated that in the brain, ZIKV preferentially infects neural stem cells (NSC), astrocytes, oligodendrocyte precursor cells, and microglia, whereas neurons are less susceptible to infection. Infection of induced pluripotent stem cell (iPSC)-derived hNPC results in cell cycle abnormalities and apoptosis. Many cellular pathways correlate with clinical pathologies following ZIKV infection such as microcephaly, congenital nervous system disorders, and epilepsy. Furthermore, ZIKV activates several inflammatory signals within infected hNPC that are implicated in innate and acquired immune responses, while CMV-infected hNPC show limited representation of these pathways. Moreover, several genes related to pathogen responses are significantly up-regulated upon ZIKV infection, but not perturbed in CMV-infected hNPC. hNPC are capable of signaling through canonic pro-inflammatory pathways following viral infection. By defining gene expression profiles, new factors in the pathogenesis of ZIKV have been identified which could help develop new therapeutic strategies [32]. hNPC are responsible for populating the developing central nervous system (CNS) with neurons and glia. Neural progenitor dysfunction can lead to severe birth defects, namely, lissencephaly, microcephaly, and cognitive deficits. ZIKV isolates from Asian and African lineages displayed lineage-specific replication kinetics, cytopathic effects, and impacts on hNPC function and neuronal differentiation. The currently circulating ZIKV isolates exhibit a unique profile of virulence, cytopathic effect, and impaired cellular functions that likely contribute to the pathological mechanism of congenital zika syndrome (CZS). Infection with Asian-lineage ZIKV isolates impaired the proliferation and migration of hNPC, and neuron maturation. In contrast, the African-lineage infections resulted in abrupt and extensive cell death [33].

These findings indeed suggest mechanisms for microcephaly and other pathological features of infants with congenital ZIKV infection that are not explained by NSC infection alone, such as calcifications in the cortical plate. Furthermore, it has been found that blocking the glia-enriched putative viral entry receptor AXL reduces *in vitro* ZIKV infection of astrocytes, and genetic knockdown of AXL in a glial cell line nearly abolishes infection. Finally, it has been showed that the macrolide antibiotic azithromycin reduces viral proliferation and virus-induced cytopathic effects in glial cell lines and human astrocytes. Characterization of infection in the developing human brain clarifies the pathogenesis of congenital ZIKV infection and provides the basis for investigating possible therapeutic strategies to safely alleviate or prevent the most severe consequences of the epidemic [34]. In addition to the developing CNS, ZIKV has been recently shown to infect cells of the PNS, highlighting its potential to cause acute peripheral neuropathies in adults, such as GBS, in a pure motor axonal variant. Myelinating dorsal root ganglia (DRG) explants obtained from IFN-alpha/beta (IFN-α/β) receptor knock-out mice are productively infected by ZIKV. Virus replication is cytopathic in both peripheral neurons and myelinating Schwann cells, leading to myelin disruption. These results confirm and extend previous observations suggesting that the PNS is indeed a potential site of ZIKV infection, replication, and cytopathicity [35]. Moreover, vertical ZIKV infection can cause a wide spectrum of neurological manifestations that go beyond microcephaly, and even the non-microcephalic child should be followed during the first years of life, because infection may be asymptomatic or lead to neuropsicomotor delay, epilepsy, and visual abnormalities. The appropriate prospective multidisciplinary follow-up of these patients aims to understand the natural history of this new agent and to provide a better development and quality of life for them and their families [36]. But whether it can induce neurological sequelae that appear later in life remains unclear. The virus unexpectedly alters the DNA methylome of neural progenitors, astrocytes, and differentiated neurons at genes that have been implicated in the pathogenesis of a number of brain disorders, most prominently mental retardation and schizophrenia. These results suggest that ZIKV infection during fetal development could lead to a spectrum of delayed-onset neuropsychiatric complications. Scientific research on human NSC and cerebral organoids has confirmed the congenital neurotropic and neuro-destructive nature of ZIKV. However, the extent to which prenatal ZIKV infection is associated with more subtle brain alterations, such as epigenetic changes, remains ill-defined [37].

In the last few years, genomic and molecular investigations have established a remarkable progress on the pathogenic mechanisms of ZIKV infection using *in vitro* and *in vivo* models [38]. Numerous experimental approaches have been taken to address how the virus can cross the placenta, alter normal fetal development, and disrupt specific cellular functions. Many areas concerning the mechanisms of transmission, especially from mother to fetus, are largely unknown but demand further research. Several promising new studies provide insight into possible mechanisms of transmission, different cell types affected, and immune responses towards the virus. By aiming to better understand the processes behind altered fetal neuronal development due to ZIKV infection, the hope is to find ways to increase protection of the fetus and prevent congenital abnormalities such as microcephaly. As ZIKV infection is spreading to increasingly more areas and bringing harmful outcomes and birth defects with it, it is imperative to identify the mechanisms of transmitting this infectious agent, consider different genetic backgrounds of hosts and strain types, and navigate methods to protect those affected from the detrimental effects of this newly emerging virus [39]. A major difficulty in management of ZIKV disease is that most infections are asymptomatic and the diagnostic methods are not ideal, making both diagnosis and ascertainment of timing of infection problematic. Understanding of the mechanisms of ZIKV-host interaction at the cellular level will contribute crucial insights into the development of ZIKV therapeutics and vaccines. Several different types of vaccines are in development. Large studies are ongoing to determine the risk and total spectrum of anomalies based on the timing of infection and other environmental exposures [40-43].

EPIDEMIOLOGY

Since many persons with mild ZIKV disease are asymptomatic and might not seek care, it is difficult to estimate the actual incidence of ZIKV infection. Arbovirus infections were at first of public health interest in East Africa, where a very widespread epidemic of o'nyong-nyong fever was reported in 1959-60 and where the threat of yellow fever, present in neighboring areas such as Ethiopia, remains. The prevalence of arbovirus infection varies markedly from area to area in Africa. Yellow fever antibodies in the coastal area must be due either to vaccination or to cross-reactions with other group-B arboviruses [44]. Serological studies of persons infected with yellow fever during the 1970 epidemic in Okwoga District, Nigeria, indicated that epidemic yellow fever occurred despite a high prevalence of pre-existing group-B arbovirus immunity, which increased with age. The viruses involved were primarily DENV, Wesselsbron Virus (WESSV), and ZIKV [45]. Mosquito and sentinel animal surveillance studies have demonstrated that ZIKV is endemic to Africa and Southeast Asia. In June 2007, an epidemic of relatively mild disease characterized by fever, rash, arthralgia, and conjunctivitis associated with ZIKV was detected in Yap State, Federated States of Micronesia, in the southwestern Pacific Ocean, where hundreds of dengue-like syndromes were reported [46]. This was the first time that ZIKV was detected outside of Africa and Asia. Then, in 2013-2014, it was reported in New Caledonia and French Polynesia, where the first neurological effects were observed. The emergence of ZIKV outside of its previously known geographic range prompted awareness of the potential for ZIKV to spread to other Pacific Islands and the Americas [47-49].

A recent study indicated the existence of three geographically distinct viral lineages. Although ZIKV has been known to circulate in both Africa and Asia since at least the 1950s, little is known about the genetic relationships between geographically distinct virus strains. Moreover, the geographic origin of the strains responsible for the epidemic that occurred on Yap Island in 2007, and a 2010 pediatric case in Cambodia, has not been determined. The basal position of the ZIKV strain isolated in Malaysia in 1966 suggests that the recent outbreak in Micronesia was initiated by a strain from Southeast Asia. Because ZIKV infection in humans produces an acute febrile illness that clinically resembles dengue fever and many other tropical infectious diseases, it is likely greatly misdiagnosed and under-reported [50, 51]. Yellow fever, zika fever, and dengue, all of which are major human diseases found in tropical regions of the globe, are zoonoses with a transmission cycle that involves primates as reservoirs and mosquitoes of the genus *Aedes* as vectors. The recent upsurge of urban epidemics of yellow fever, zika fever, and dengue has involved human-to-human transmission with mosquitoes as the vector [52]. Clinical descriptions of chikungunya fever have been performed in the American outbreak observing that fever, polyarthalgia, myalgia, and rash are the most common symptoms in the acute phase, while chronic arthralgia has persisted in 37-90% of small cohorts. The Asian origin of American strains of CHIKV and ZIKV evidences a dissemination route in common and both are being transmitted by *Aedes aegypti*. Regarding zika fever, the association of congenital malformations with previous ZIKV exposure of pregnant women and potential sexual transmission of ZIKV are the most important discoveries in the New World. Massive outbreaks of chikungunya fever in 2014 and then followed by zika fever epidemics of lower magnitude in the next year throughout the American continent have their origins in Asia but may have used Pacific Islands as a path of dissemination. Reports of chronic arthralgia have been little described in the continent and more research is needed to measure the economic and health impact in patients who contracted CHIKV before. On the contrary, zika is menacing newborns' health because of its link with congenital microcephaly and sexual health by prolonged presence of viral particles in semen and urine [53].

As we have seen, before 2007, only sporadic human disease cases were reported from Countries in Africa and Asia. In 2007, the first documented outbreak of ZIKV disease was reported in Yap State; 73% of the population aged at least three years is estimated to have been infected. Subsequent outbreaks occurred in Southeast Asia and the Western Pacific, on the heels of a CHIKV epidemic in the Americas that began in 2013. In 2014, the WHO reported the first local transmission of ZIKV in the Region of the Americas on Easter Island, Chile, and in Northeast Brazil in May 2015. The virus was likely introduced in Brazil from competing athletes from French Polynesia and other Countries that participated in a competition there, from where it has rapidly expanded in the continent; the first case in Mexico was detected in October 2015, the first cases of local transmission have just been reported in Florida, and in the following months has spread also across southern states of US, including the Commonwealth of Puerto Rico and the US Virgin Islands (USVI). In May 2015, the Pan American Health Organization (PAHO), which serves as the Regional Office for the Americas (RAM) for the WHO, issued an alert regarding the first confirmed ZIKV infection in Brazil. In October 2015, in Pernambuco, Brazil, an increase in the number of newborns with microcephaly was reported. Women delivering in October would have been in the first trimester of pregnancy during the peak of a zika epidemic in March. By the end of 2015, 4,180 cases of suspected microcephaly had been reported [54]. In Salvador, Brazil, outbreaks of acute exanthematous illness (AEI) attributed to ZIKV, GBS, and microcephaly occurred in 2015. Temporal correlations and time lags between these outbreaks have been investigated to identify a common link between them by using epidemic curves and time series cross-correlations. Number of GBS cases peaked after a lag of five to nine weeks from the AEI peak. Number of suspected cases of microcephaly peaked after a lag of 30-33 weeks from the AEI peak, which corresponded to time of potential infections of pregnant mothers during the first trimester. These findings support the association of GBS and microcephaly with ZIKV infection and provide evidence for a temporal relationship between timing of arboviral infection of pregnant women during the first trimester and birth outcome [55].

Neurological disorders among zika patients were similar in Brazil and French Polynesia, but a causal link is not established. Incidence of zika infection in pregnant women is not known. In Brazil, during the zika outbreak the incidence of microcephaly increased more than 20 times. Among 35 infants with microcephaly, born from women suspected to have zika infection during pregnancy in Northeast Brazil, 74% of the mothers reported rash during the first and second trimester and no exposure to other potentially teratogenic agents [56-58]. During October 12th, 2015-September 10th, 2016, the Haitian Ministry of Public Health and Population (MOPHP) detected 3,036 suspected cases of ZIKV infection in the general population, 22 suspected cases of ZIKV disease among pregnant women, 13 suspected cases of GBS, and 29 suspected cases of zika-associated congenital microcephaly. Nineteen (0.6%) patients with suspected ZIKV disease, residing in Ouest (10 patients), Artibonite (six), and Centre (three) administrative departments, have been confirmed by laboratory testing, including two among pregnant women and 17 in the general population [59]. Air, land, and sea transportation can facilitate rapid spread of infectious diseases. New York City (NYC) is home to a large number of persons who travel frequently to areas with active ZIKV transmission, including immigrants from these areas. In November 2015, the NYC Department of Health and Mental Hygiene (DOHMH) began developing and implementing plans for managing ZIKV and on February 1st, 2016, activated its Incident Command System (ICS). During January 1st-June 17th, 2016, DOHMH coordinated diagnostic laboratory testing for 3,605 persons with travel-associated exposure, 182 (5.0%) of whom had confirmed ZIKV infection. Twenty (11.0%) confirmed patients were pregnant at the time of diagnosis. In addition, two cases of ZIKV-associated GBS were diagnosed. DOHMH's response has focused on:

1) identifying and diagnosing suspected cases;
2) educating the public and medical providers about ZIKV risks, transmission, and prevention strategies, particularly in areas with large populations of immigrants from areas with ongoing ZIKV transmission;
3) monitoring pregnant women with ZIKV infection and their fetuses and infants;
4) detecting local mosquito-borne transmission through both human and mosquito surveillance; and
5) modifying existing *Culex* mosquito control measures by targeting *Aedes* species of mosquitoes through the use of larvicides and adulticides [60].

Recent outbreaks of ZIKV disease in the Pacific Islands and the Region of the Americas and the Caribbean, including Haiti, have identified new modes of transmission and clinical manifestations. During December 2015-January 2016, the American Samoa Department of Health (ASDoH) detected through surveillance an increase in the number of cases of acute febrile rash illness. Concurrently, a case of laboratory-confirmed ZIKV infection was reported in a traveler returning to New Zealand from American Samoa. In the absence of local laboratory capacity to test for ZIKV, ASDoH initiated arboviral disease control measures, including public education and vector source reduction campaigns. On February 1st, CDC staff members were deployed to American Samoa to assist ASDoH with testing and surveillance efforts [61]. In December 2015, the Ministry of Health (MoH) estimated that 440,000-1,300,000 suspected cases of ZIKV disease had occurred in Brazil in 2015. On December 31st, 2015,

Puerto Rico Department of Health (PRDH) reported the first locally acquired case of ZIKV disease in a jurisdiction of the US in a patient from southeastern Puerto Rico, with the index patient reporting symptom onset on November 23rd, 2015. During November 23rd, 2015-January 28th, 2016, passive and enhanced surveillance for ZIKV disease identified 30 laboratory-confirmed cases. Most (93%) patients resided in eastern Puerto Rico or the San Juan metropolitan area. The most frequently reported signs and symptoms were rash (77%), myalgia (77%), arthralgia (73%), and fever (73%). Three (10%) patients were hospitalized. One case occurred in a patient hospitalized for GBS, and one occurred in a pregnant woman. Because the most common mosquito vector of ZIKV, *Aedes aegypti*, is present throughout Puerto Rico, ZIKV was expected to continue to spread across the island. The public health response in Puerto Rico is being coordinated by PRDH with assistance from CDC. By January 20th, 2016, locally-transmitted cases had been reported to the PAHO from Puerto Rico and 19 other Countries or territories in the Americas. Further spread to other Countries in the region has been monitored closely [62]. During November 1st, 2015-April 14th, 2016, a total of 6,157 specimens from suspected ZIKV-infected patients were evaluated by the PRDH and CDC Dengue Branch (DB), which is located in San Juan, Puerto Rico, and 683 (11%) had laboratory evidence of current or recent ZIKV infection by one or more tests: reverse transcription-polymerase chain reaction (RT-PCR) or immunoglobulin M (IgM) enzyme-linked immunosorbent assay (ELISA). ZIKV-infected patients resided in 50 (64%) of 78 municipalities in Puerto Rico. Median age was 34 years (range = 35-89 years). The most frequently reported signs and symptoms were rash (74%), myalgia (68%), headache (63%), fever (63%), and arthralgia (63%). There were 65 (10%) symptomatic pregnant women who tested positive by RT-PCR or IgM ELISA. A total of 17 (2%) patients required hospitalization, including five (1%) patients with suspected GBS. One (<1%) patient died after developing severe thrombocytopenia. The public health response to the outbreak has included increased laboratory capacity to test for ZIKV infection (including blood donor screening), implementation of enhanced surveillance systems, and prevention activities focused on pregnant women. Vector control activities include indoor and outdoor residual spraying and reduction of mosquito breeding environments focused around pregnant women's homes [63]. During November 1st, 2015-July 7th, 2016, a total of 23,487 persons were evaluated by PRDH and CDC DB for ZIKV infection, including asymptomatic pregnant women and persons with signs or symptoms consistent with ZIKV disease or suspected GBS; 5,582 (24%) confirmed and presumptive ZIKV cases were identified. Persons with ZIKV infection were residents of 77 (99%) of Puerto Rico's 78 municipalities. During 2016, the percentage of positive ZIKV infection cases among symptomatic males and non-pregnant females who were tested increased from 14% in February to 64% in June. Among 9,343 pregnant women tested, 672 had confirmed or presumptive ZIKV infection, including 441 (66%) symptomatic women and 231 (34%) asymptomatic women. One patient died after developing severe thrombocytopenia. Evidence of ZIKV infection or recent unspecified Flavivirus infection was detected in 21 patients with confirmed GBS [64]. During November 1st, 2015-October 20th, 2016, 62,500 suspected ZIKV disease cases were reported to the PRDH; 29,345 (47%) were confirmed by RT-PCR testing, or were presumptively diagnosed based on serological testing. The highest incidence among confirmed or presumptive cases occurred among persons aged 20-29 years (1,150 cases per 100,000 residents). Among 28,219 (96.2%) non-pregnant patients with confirmed or presumptive ZIKV disease, incidence was higher among women (936 per 100,000 population) than men (576 per 100,000) for all age groups ≥20 years, and the majority (61%) of reported ZIKV disease cases occurred in females. Among suspected ZIKV disease cases in non-pregnant adults aged ≥40 years, the percentage that tested positive among females (52%) was higher than that among males (47%) ($p<0.01$). Reasons for the higher incidence of ZIKV disease among women aged ≥20 years are not known; serosurveys of persons living near confirmed ZIKV disease cases might help to elucidate these findings. Residents of and travelers to Puerto Rico should remove or cover standing water, practice mosquito abatement, employ mosquito bite avoidance behaviors, take precautions to reduce the risk for sexual transmission, and seek medical care for any acute illness with rash or fever [65]. Clinicians should report all cases of microcephaly, GBS, and suspected ZIKV disease. Other adverse reproductive outcomes, including fetal demise associated with ZIKV infection, should be reported. To avoid infection with ZIKV, residents of and visitors to these regions, particularly pregnant women, should strictly follow steps to avoid mosquito bites, including wearing pants and long-sleeved shirts, using permethrin-treated clothing and gear, using an Environmental Protection Agency (EPA)-registered insect repellent, and ensuring that windows and doors have intact screens [66].

During January 1st, 2015-February 26th, 2016, a total of 116 residents of 33 US and the District of Columbia (DC) had laboratory evidence of recent ZIKV infection based on testing performed at CDC. Cases include one congenital infection and 115 persons who reported recent travel to areas with active ZIKV transmission (n = 110) or sexual contact with such a traveler (n = 5). All 115 patients had clinical illness, with the most common signs and symptoms being rash (98%; n = 113), fever (82%; 94), and arthralgia (66%; 76) [67, 68]. As of September 3rd, 2016, a total of 2,382 confirmed and probable cases of ZIKV disease with symptom onset during January 1st-July 31st, 2016, had been reported from 48 of 50 US and the DC. Most cases (2,354; 99%) were travel-associated, with either direct travel or an epidemiological link to a traveler to a ZIKV-affected area. Twenty-eight (1%) cases were reported as locally acquired, including 26 associated with mosquito-borne transmission, one acquired in a laboratory, and one with an unknown mode of transmission. In 2016, a total of 5,168 non-congenital ZIKV disease cases were reported from US and the DC. Most cases (4,897, 95%) were in travelers returning from ZIKV-affected areas. A total of 224 (4%) cases were acquired through presumed local mosquito-borne transmission, and 47 (1%) were acquired by other routes. It is important that providers in the US continue to test symptomatic patients who live in or recently traveled to areas with ongoing ZIKV transmission or had unprotected sex with someone who lives in or traveled to those areas. All pregnant women and their partners should take measures to prevent ZIKV infection during pregnancy. ZIKV disease should be considered in patients with compatible clinical signs or symptoms who traveled to or reside in areas with ongoing ZIKV transmission or who had unprotected sex with someone who traveled to those areas. Health care providers should continue to educate patients, especially pregnant women, about the importance of avoiding infection with ZIKV, and all pregnant women should be assessed for possible ZIKV exposure at each prenatal visit [69-71].

On February 1st, 2016, the WHO declared the occurrence of ZIKV-related microcephaly clusters and other neurological disorders to be a PHEIC and that, although not yet scientifically proven, the link between the virus and growing numbers of microcephaly cases was "strongly suspected," and now talks about a ZIKV pandemic. However, the causal relationship between zika and microcephaly is not universally accepted. Although ZIKV infections may explain many cases of brain damage in newborns, it may not be the only cause. We need a clear association between confirmed cases of zika infections in pregnant women and microcephaly in newborns. Certainly, the ZIKV, as many other viruses, has the capacity to induce severe cerebral lesions in fetuses of women infected during the first months of pregnancy. Moreover, more than 80% of cases of craniostenosys that verisimilarly took place in Brazil from September 2015 up to now were registered in few states of northeastern Brazil, where peaks of this malformation were registered several years before the appearance of ZIKV. In addition, in none of the 60 Countries where ZIKV is epidemiologically active an increase of the incidence of microcephaly had been reported. Despite initial skepticism regarding the causal association of the ZIKV epidemic and birth defects, extensive basic and clinical research evidence has now confirmed this relationship [72]. However, data on the epidemiology and clinical findings of laboratory-confirmed ZIKV disease remain limited. Because ZIKV is a relatively new infection with several transmission routes that include mosquito bites, sexual, and possibly blood-related, a parallel between the zika epidemic and the acquired immunodeficiency syndrome (AIDS) epidemic for issues that relate particularly to pregnancy and epidemic response can be made. However, the viruses are different and the pathophysiology and disease manifestation are also different. Nevertheless, parallels between the zika and the Human

Immunodeficiency Virus (HIV)/AIDS epidemics, particularly in relation to pregnancy, can be established. Lessons and successes from the HIV/AIDS epidemic control efforts can guide us towards comprehensive approaches to improve the health of women and infants at risk for zika [73].

The association between maternal ZIKV infection and adverse fetal and reproductive outcomes, including microcephaly, prompted CDC to issue a level two alert travel notice for the 37 Countries and three US territories (at the national and territorial level) that have reported recent ZIKV transmission as of March 11th, 2016. An estimated 216.3 million passenger journeys by air, land, and sea are made annually to the US from areas with local ZIKV transmission (as of March 8th). The destination states with the largest numbers of arrivals were Texas (by land) and Florida (by air and sea). An estimated 51.7 million passenger journeys were made by women of childbearing age and an estimated 2.3 million were made by pregnant women. Travel volume analyses provide important information that can be used to effectively target public health interventions as well as direct public health resources and efforts at local, regional, and Country-specific levels [74]. The vector is widely distributed in South America and control measures are the most effective means for prevention, not only of ZIKV, but also DENV and CHIKV [75]. In addition to mosquito bite precautions for all travelers, CDC advises that pregnant women postpone travel to affected Countries and US territories. Within a nation's borders, ecological characteristics, which determine the distribution of mosquito vectors, can vary considerably. CDC conducted a spatial analysis, focusing on the probability of occurrence of *Aedes aegypti*, to support the demarcation for sub-national travel alerts. Based on results of this analysis, travel that is limited to elevations higher than 2,000 m (6,562 ft) above sea level is considered to have minimal (approximately 1%) likelihood for mosquito-borne ZIKV transmission, even within countries reporting active transmission. Women who are pregnant should avoid travel to elevations <2,000 m in countries with active ZIKV transmission [76-82].

ZIKV originated and continues to circulate in a sylvatic transmission cycle between non-human primate hosts and arboreal mosquitoes in tropical Africa. Recently, ZIKV invaded the Americas, where it poses a threat to human health, especially to pregnant women and their infants. Brazil is home to multiple species of primates and mosquitoes potentially capable of ZIKV transmission, though direct assessment of host competence (ability to mount viremia sufficient to infect a feeding mosquito) and vector competence (ability to become infected with ZIKV and disseminate and transmit upon subsequent feedings) of New World species is lacking. Modeling reveals a high probability of establishment of sylvatic ZIKV across a large range of biologically plausible parameters. Probability of establishment is dependent on host and vector population sizes, host birthrates, and ZIKV force of infection. Research on the host competence of New World monkeys or other small mammals to ZIKV, on vector competence of New World *Aedes*, *Sabethes*, and *Hemagogus* mosquitoes for ZIKV, and on the geographic range of potential New World hosts and vectors is urgently needed. A sylvatic cycle of ZIKV would make future elimination efforts in the Americas practically impossible, and paints a dire picture for the epidemiology of ZIKV and our ability to end the ongoing outbreak of CZS [83]. Mechanistic models of disease transmission can be used to forecast trajectories and likely disease burden but are currently hampered by substantial uncertainty on the epidemiology of the disease (e.g., the role of asymptomatic transmission, generation interval, incubation period, and key drivers). When insight is limited, phenomenological models provide a starting point for estimation of key transmission parameters, such as the reproduction number, and forecasts of epidemic impact. Phenomenological models represent promising tools to generate early forecasts of epidemic impact particularly in the context of substantial uncertainty in epidemiological parameters. Findings underscore the need to treat the reproduction number as a dynamic quantity even during the early growth phase, and emphasize the sensitivity of reproduction number estimates to assumptions on the generation interval distribution [84-86].

Mosquito-borne diseases pose a threat to individual health and population health on both a local and a global level. The threat is even more exaggerated during disasters, whether man-made or environmental. Education and training are instrumental in controlling the outbreak, and early detection can be life-saving [87]. This epidemic currently continues unabated. The explosive nature of recent outbreaks and concerning links to GBS and microcephaly are incompletely understood. Also unknown is the relative importance of sexual transmission of ZIKV and asymptomatic ZIKV infections to the overall burden of transmission. The limited understanding of ZIKV presents an enormous challenge for responses to this rapidly emerging threat to human health [88-94].

Obstetric and Pediatric Issues

It has been recognized for centuries that pregnant women have unique susceptibilities to many infectious diseases that predispose them to untoward outcomes compared with the general adult population. It is thought a combination of adaptive alterations in immunity to allow for the fetal allograft combined with changes in anatomy and physiology accompanying pregnancy underlie these susceptibilities. Emerging infectious diseases are defined as those whose incidence in humans has increased in the past two decades or threaten to increase in the near future. The past decade alone has witnessed many such outbreaks, each with its own unique implications for pregnant women and their unborn fetuses as well as lessons for the health care community regarding response and mitigation. Examples of such outbreaks include, but are not limited to, severe acute respiratory syndrome (SARS), the 2009 A Hemagglutinin 1 and Neuraminidase 1 Virus (H1N1) pandemic influenza, Ebola Virus (EBOV), and, most recently, ZIKV. Although each emerging pathogen has unique features requiring specific considerations, there are many underlying principles that are shared in the recognition, communication, and mitigation of such infectious outbreaks. Some of these key principles include disease-specific delineation of transmission dynamics, understanding of pathogen-specific effects on both mothers and fetuses, and advance planning and contemporaneous management that prioritize communication among public health experts, clinicians, and patients. The productive and effective working collaboration among the CDC, the

American College of Obstetricians and Gynecologists (ACOG), and the Society for Maternal-Fetal Medicine (SMFM) has been a key partnership in the successful communication and management of such outbreaks for women's health care providers and patients alike. Going forward, the knowledge gained over the past decade will undoubtedly continue to inform future responses and will serve to optimize the education and care given to pregnant women in the face of current and future emerging infectious disease outbreaks [95]. Congenital infectious diseases, transmitted during the course of pregnancy, are estimated to affect nearly one in every 100 births worldwide. These infections may be associated with fetal and infant adverse health outcomes, due to congenital malformations caused by *in utero* transmission of the infectious organism itself (as is the case with CMV, toxoplasmosis, syphilis, and ZIKV), or due to chronic infection in the infant (as is the case with HIV and Hepatitis B Virus [HBV] and Hepatitis C Virus [HCV]). In addition, children who are exposed, yet uninfected, may still suffer from the consequences of exposure to infectious pathogens or to the drugs given to treat pregnant women and prevent *in utero* transmission (as may be the case with HIV infection) [96]. The recent association between ZIKV infection during pregnancy and fetal microcephaly has led to a renewed interest in the mechanisms by which vertically transmitted micro-organisms reach the fetus and cause congenital disease. Based on our current understanding of ZIKV pathogenesis and the developmental defects that are caused by fetal ZIKV infection, ZIKV should be considered a TORCH pathogen and future research and public health measures should be planned and implemented accordingly [97]. The acronym TORCH is used to refer to congenital infections, such as toxoplasmosis, other infections (such as syphilis, Varicella-Zoster Virus [VZV], and Parvovirus B19), CMV, and HSV. Three of the original TORCH agents are associated with an appreciable incidence of congenital microcephaly: CMV, RuV, and *Toxoplasma gondii*. The pathology of congenital microcephaly is characterized by neurotropic infectious agents that involve the fetal nervous system, leading to brain destruction with calcifications, microcephaly, sensorineural hearing loss, and ophthalmological abnormalities. The inflammatory reaction induced by these four agents has an important role in pathogenesis. Specific epidemiological factors, such as first and early second trimester maternal infection, and the manifestations of congenital infection in the infant, shed some light on the pathogenesis [98]. The classic findings in patients with TORCH infections include rash in the mother during pregnancy and ocular findings in the newborn. ZIKV has emerged as an important worldwide congenital infection. It fits well with other congenital TORCH infections since there is a rash in the mother and there are commonly ocular abnormalities in the newborn. TORCH infections are recognized to have neurological effects, such as ventriculomegaly, intraventricular adhesions, subependymal cysts, intracerebral calcifications, and microcephaly; however, ZIKV is intensely neurotropic. In fact, it targets hNPC, leading to a more severe spectrum of CNS abnormalities than is typically seen in other TORCH infections, while relatively sparing the other organ systems. Awareness of imaging features of common congenital infections may facilitate early diagnosis and may, at times, lead to prompt initiation of therapy [99].

By September 2015, reports of an increase in the number of infants born with microcephaly in ZIKV-affected areas began to emerge, and ZIKV RNA was identified in the amniotic fluid of two women whose fetuses had been found to have microcephaly by prenatal ultrasound. More than 4,700 suspected cases of microcephaly were reported from mid-2015 through January 2016, many of which occurred in infants born to women who lived in or had visited areas where ZIKV transmission was occurring [100]. Microcephaly surveillance was enhanced in late 2015 by implementing a more sensitive case definition. Based on the peak number of reported cases of microcephaly, and assuming an average estimated pregnancy duration of 38 weeks in Brazil, the first trimester of pregnancy coincided with reports of cases of febrile rash illness compatible with ZIKV disease in pregnant women in Bahia, Paraíba, and Pernambuco states, supporting an association between ZIKV infection during early pregnancy and the occurrence of microcephaly [101]. The Brazil MoH established a task force to investigate the possible association of microcephaly with ZIKV infection during pregnancy and a registry for incident microcephaly cases (head circumference at least two standard deviations [SD] below the mean for sex and gestational age at birth) and pregnancy outcomes among women suspected to have had ZIKV infection during pregnancy. Among a cohort of 35 infants with microcephaly born during August-October 2015 in eight of Brazil's 26 states and reported to the registry, the mothers of all 35 had lived in or visited ZIKV-affected areas during pregnancy, 25 (71%) infants had severe microcephaly (head circumference more than three SD below the mean for sex and gestational age), 17 (49%) had at least one neurological abnormality, and among 27 infants who had neuroimaging studies, all had abnormalities. Tests for other congenital infections were negative. All infants had a lumbar puncture as part of the evaluation and CSF samples were sent to a reference laboratory in Brazil for ZIKV testing [102]. The link with brain defect, which has been detected mainly in some areas of Brazil, is supported by the following evidence:

1) ZIKV transmission from infected pregnant women to their fetuses; and
2) the potential of ZIKV to determine a specific congenital fetal syndrome characterized by abnormalities involving primarily the developing brain and eye.

In particular, the risk of transmission and congenital disease appears to be restricted to mother's infection during the first trimester of pregnancy. Among brain defects, microcephaly, brain calcifications, and ventriculomegaly are the most frequent abnormalities of the CNS detected so far [103]. About 60% to 70% of mothers report rash during pregnancy, mainly in the first trimester. Principal features are microcephaly, facial disproportionality, *cutis girata*, hypertonia/spasticity, hyperreflexia, and irritability; abnormal neuroimages include calcifications, ventriculomegaly, and lissencephaly. Hearing and visual abnormalities may be present. Preliminary data suggest that severe congenital abnormalities are linked to ZIKV infection. Cases have severe abnormalities, and although sharing many characteristics with congenital abnormalities associated with other viral infections, abnormalities presumably linked to ZIKV may have distinguishing characteristics. These severe neurological abnormalities may result in marked mental retardation and motor disabilities for many surviving offspring [104]. In most studies, ZIKV seems related to congenital ocular lesions and most mothers reported mild symptoms during the first trimester of pregnancy. Five fundus patterns were seen most often: macular chorioretinal atrophy, chorioretinal atrophy elsewhere, focal pigmentary changes in the macular region, optic nerve abnormalities, and combined types. A few studies have suggested that ZIKV might damage the anterior segment of these babies' eyes. Few reports have described the ocular complications seen in adults during the acute infection, including conjunctivitis, iridocyclitis, and chorioretinitis. Infants with CZS might have vision-threatening fundus abnormalities. Although the full spectrum of ocular lesions caused by ZIKV infection is not yet determined, a distinctive new disease has been observed. Recognition of these lesions can help ensure appropriate etiological evaluation and clinical investigation to define the range of anomalies in an affected infant and determine essential follow-up and ongoing care [105-107]. Hearing loss associated with other congenital viral infections is well described; however, little is known about hearing loss in infants with congenital ZIKV infection. A retrospective assessment of a series of 70 infants aged from zero to 10 months with microcephaly and laboratory evidence of ZIKV infection was conducted by the Hospital Agamenon Magalhães in Brazil and partners. The infants were enrolled during November 2015-May 2016 and had screening and diagnostic hearing tests. Five (7%) infants had sensorineural hearing loss, all of whom had severe microcephaly; however, one child was tested after receiving treatment with an ototoxic antibiotic. If this child is excluded, the prevalence of sensorineural hearing loss was 5.8% (four of 69), which is similar to that seen in association with other congenital viral infections. Additional information is needed to understand the prevalence and spectrum of hearing loss in children with congenital ZIKV infection; all infants born to women with evidence of ZIKV infection during pregnancy should have their hearing tested, including infants who appear normal at birth [108].

Population-based birth defects surveillance systems are critical to monitor all infants and fetuses with birth defects potentially related to ZIKV infection, regardless of known exposure or laboratory evidence of ZIKV infection during pregnancy. To inform microcephaly surveillance efforts and assess ascertainment sources, the New York State Department of Health (NYSDOH) and the NYC Department of Health and Mental Hygiene (DOHMH) sought to determine the prevalence of microcephaly in New York during 2013-2015, before known importation of ZIKV infections. Suspected newborn microcephaly diagnoses were identified from:

1) reports submitted by birth hospitals in response to a request; and
2) queries of a hospital administrative discharge database for newborn microcephaly diagnoses.

Anthropometric measurements, maternal demographics, and pregnancy characteristics were abstracted from newborn records from both sources. Diagnoses were classified using microcephaly case definitions developed by CDC and the National Birth Defects Prevention Network (NBDPN). During 2013-2015, 284 newborns in New York met the case definition for severe congenital microcephaly (prevalence = 4.2 per 10,000 live births). Most newborns with severe congenital microcephaly were identified by both sources; 263 (93%) were identified through hospital requests and 256 (90%) were identified through administrative discharge data. The proportions of newborns with severe congenital microcephaly who were black (30%) or Hispanic (31%) were higher than the observed proportions of black (15%) or Hispanic (23%) infants among New York live births. Fifty-eight percent of newborns with severe congenital microcephaly were born to mothers with pregnancy complications or who had *in utero* or perinatal infections or teratogenic exposures, genetic disorders, or family histories of birth defects [109]. In November 2015, the Brazilian MoH declared the ZIKV outbreak a public health emergency after an increase in microcephaly cases was reported in the Northeast Region of the Country. During 2015-2016, 15 states in Brazil with laboratory-confirmed ZIKV transmission reported an increase in birth prevalence of microcephaly (2.8 cases per 10,000 live births), significantly exceeding prevalence in four states without confirmed transmission (0.6 per 10,000). Although children with microcephaly and laboratory evidence of ZIKV infection have been described in early infancy, their subsequent health and development have not been well characterized, constraining planning for the care and support of these children and their families. The Brazilian MoH, the State Health Secretariat of Paraíba, and CDC collaborated on a follow-up investigation of the health and development of children in northeastern Brazil who were reported to national surveillance with microcephaly at birth. Nineteen children with microcephaly at birth and laboratory evidence of ZIKV infection were assessed through clinical evaluations, caregiver interviews, and review of medical records. At follow-up (ages 19-24 months), most of these children had severe motor impairment, seizure disorders, hearing and vision abnormalities, and sleep difficulties. Children with microcephaly and laboratory evidence of ZIKV infection have severe functional limitations and will require specialized care from clinicians and caregivers as they age [110]. Initial descriptions of the effects of *in utero* ZIKV infection centered prominently on the finding of congenital microcephaly. To assess the possibility of clinical presentations that do not include congenital microcephaly, a retrospective assessment of 13 infants from the Brazilian states of Pernambuco and Ceará with normal head size at birth and laboratory evidence of congenital ZIKV infection was conducted. All infants had brain abnormalities on neuroimaging consistent with CZS, including decreased brain volume, ventriculomegaly, subcortical calcifications, and cortical malformations. The earliest evaluation occurred on the second day of life. Among all infants, head growth was documented to have decelerated as early as five months of age, and 11 infants had microcephaly. These findings provide evidence that among infants with prenatal exposure to ZIKV, the absence of microcephaly at birth does not exclude congenital ZIKV infection or the presence of zika-related brain and other abnormalities. These findings support the recommendation for comprehensive medical and developmental follow-up of infants exposed to ZIKV prenatally. Early neuroimaging might identify brain abnormalities related to congenital zika infection even among infants with a normal head circumference [111]. The WHO stated in March 2016 that there was scientific consensus that ZIKV was a cause of the neurological disorder GBS and of microcephaly and other congenital brain abnormalities based on rapid evidence assessments. Decisions about causality require systematic assessment to guide public health actions. WHO convened a multidisciplinary panel of experts who reached consensus statements to update the WHO position on causality. The expert panel concluded that:

1) the most likely explanation of available evidence from outbreaks of ZIKV infection and clusters of microcephaly is that ZIKV infection during pregnancy is a cause of congenital brain abnormalities, including microcephaly; and
2) the most likely explanation of available evidence from outbreaks of ZIKV infection and GBS is that ZIKV infection is a trigger of GBS.

The expert panel recognized that ZIKV alone may not be sufficient to cause either congenital brain abnormalities or GBS but agreed that the evidence was sufficient to recommend increased public health measures [112]. The establishment of a comprehensive surveillance system to monitor pregnant women with ZIKV infection will provide data to further elucidate the full range of potential outcomes for fetuses and infants of mothers with asymptomatic and symptomatic ZIKV infection during pregnancy. In February 2016, ZIKV disease and congenital ZIKV infections became nationally notifiable conditions in the US. Cases in pregnant women with laboratory evidence of ZIKV infection who have either:

1) symptomatic infection; or
2) asymptomatic infection with diagnosed complications of pregnancy;

can be reported as cases of ZIKV disease to ArboNET, CDC's national arboviral diseases surveillance system. Under existing interim guidelines from the Council for State and Territorial Epidemiologists (CSTE), asymptomatic ZIKV infections in pregnant women who do not have known pregnancy complications are not reportable. ArboNET does not currently include pregnancy surveillance information (e.g., gestational age or pregnancy exposures) or pregnancy outcomes. To understand the full impact of infection on the fetus and neonate, other systems are needed for reporting and active monitoring of pregnant women with laboratory evidence of possible ZIKV infection during pregnancy. Thus, in collaboration with state, local, tribal, and territorial health departments, CDC established two surveillance systems to monitor pregnancies and congenital outcomes among women with laboratory evidence of ZIKV infection in the US and territories:

1) the US Zika Pregnancy and Infant Registry (USZPIR), which monitors pregnant women residing in US and territories except Puerto Rico; and
2) the Zika Active Pregnancy Surveillance System (ZAPSS), which monitors pregnant women residing in Puerto Rico.

As of May 12th, 2016, the surveillance systems were monitoring 157 and 122 pregnant women with laboratory evidence of possible ZIKV infection from participating US and territories, respectively. Tracking and monitoring clinical presentation of ZIKV infection, all prenatal testing, and adverse consequences of ZIKV infection during pregnancy are critical to better characterize the risk for congenital infection, the performance of prenatal diagnostic testing, and the spectrum of adverse congenital outcomes. These data will improve clinical guidance, inform counseling messages for pregnant women, and facilitate planning for clinical and public health services for affected families [113]. To better understand the impact of birth defects resulting from ZIKV infection, the CDC surveillance case definition established in 2016 for birth defects potentially related to ZIKV infection was retrospectively applied to population-based birth defects surveillance data collected during 2013-2014 in three areas before the introduction of ZIKV (the pre-zika years) into the WHO's Region of the Americas. These data, from Massachusetts (2013), North Carolina (2013), and Atlanta, Georgia (2013-2014), included 747 infants and fetuses with one or more of the birth defects meeting the case definition (pre-zika prevalence = 2.86 per 1,000 live births). Brain abnormalities or microcephaly were the most frequently recorded (1.50 per 1,000), followed by neural tube defects (NTD) and other early brain malformations (0.88), eye abnormalities without mention of a brain abnormality (0.31), and other consequences of CNS dysfunction without mention of brain or eye abnormalities (0.17). During January 15th-September 22nd, 2016, the USZPIR reported 26 infants and fetuses with these same defects among 442 completed pregnancies (58.8 per 1,000) born to mothers with laboratory evidence of possible ZIKV infection during pregnancy. Although the ascertainment methods differed, this finding was approximately 20 times higher than the proportion of one or more of the same birth defects among pregnancies during the pre-zika years. These data demonstrate the importance of population-based surveillance for interpreting data about birth defects potentially related to ZIKV infection [114]. As of November 2016, the Florida Department of Health (FDH) and the CDC have confirmed more than 4,000 travel-related ZIKV infections in the US with >700 of those in Florida. There have been 139 cases of locally acquired infection, all occurring in Miami, Florida. Within the US territories (e.g., Puerto Rico, USVI), >30,000 cases of ZIKV infection have been reported. The projected number of individuals at risk for ZIKV infection in Latin America and the Caribbean (LAC) approximates five million. South Florida is an epicenter for ZIKV infection in the US and the year-round warm climate along with an abundance of mosquito vectors that can harbor the Flavivirus raise health care concerns. Federal health officials observed 899 confirmed zika-positive pregnancies and the FDH monitored 110 pregnant women with evidence of zika infection. The University of Miami/Jackson Memorial Hospital is uniquely positioned just North of downtown Miami and within the vicinity of Liberty City, Little Haiti, and Miami Beach, which are currently "hot spots" for ZIKV exposure and transmission. As the FDH works fervently to prevent a zika epidemic in the region, health care providers at the University of Miami and Jackson Memorial Hospital prepare for the clinical spectrum of ZIKV effects as well as the safe peri-operative care of the parturients and their affected newborns [115]. In Colombia, approximately 105,000 suspected cases of ZIKV disease (diagnosed based on clinical symptoms, regardless of laboratory confirmation) were reported during August 9th, 2015-November 12th, 2016, including nearly 20,000 in pregnant women. Colombia's Instituto Nacional de Salud (INS) maintains national surveillance for birth defects, including microcephaly and other CNS defects. This report provided preliminary information on cases of congenital microcephaly identified in Colombia during epidemic weeks five to 45 (January 31st-November 12th) in 2016. During this period, 476 cases of microcephaly were reported, compared with 110 cases reported during the same period in 2015. The temporal association between reported ZIKV infections and the occurrence of microcephaly, with the peak number of reported microcephaly cases occurring approximately 24 weeks after the peak of the ZIKV disease outbreak, provides evidence suggesting that the period of highest risk is during the first trimester of pregnancy and early in the second trimester of pregnancy. Microcephaly prevalence increased more than fourfold overall during the study period, from 2.1 per 10,000 live births in 2015 to 9.6 in 2016. Ongoing population-based birth defects surveillance is essential for monitoring the impact of ZIKV infection during pregnancy on birth defects prevalence and measuring the success in preventing ZIKV infection and its consequences, including microcephaly [116]. On November 28th, 2016, the Texas Department of State Health Services (DSHS) reported its first confirmed case of local mosquito-borne ZIKV transmission in the city of Brownsville, located in South Texas along the US-Mexico border. On January 1st, 2017, Texas DSHS established enhanced surveillance to identify women with laboratory evidence of possible ZIKV infection during pregnancy and suspected cases of ZIKV-associated birth defects among completed pregnancies [117]. Another report included an analysis of completed pregnancies (which include live births and pregnancy losses, regardless of gestational age) in the 50 US and the DC with laboratory evidence of possible recent ZIKV infection reported to the USZPIR from January 15th to December 27th, 2016. Birth defects potentially associated with ZIKV infection during pregnancy include brain abnormalities and/or microcephaly, eye abnormalities, other consequences of CNS dysfunction, and NTD and other early brain malformations. During the analysis period, 1,297 pregnant women in 44 states were reported to the USZPIR. ZIKV-associated birth defects were reported for 51 (5%) of the 972 fetuses/infants from completed pregnancies with laboratory evidence of possible recent ZIKV infection (95% CI = 4-7%); the proportion was higher when restricted to pregnancies with laboratory-confirmed ZIKV infection (24/250 completed pregnancies [10%, 95% CI = 7-14%]). Birth defects were reported in 15% (95% CI = 8-26%) of fetuses/infants of completed pregnancies with confirmed ZIKV infection in the first trimester. Among 895 liveborn infants from pregnancies with possible recent ZIKV infection, postnatal neuroimaging was reported for 221 (25%), and ZIKV testing of at least one infant specimen was reported for 585 (65%). These findings highlight why pregnant women should avoid ZIKV exposure. Because the full clinical spectrum of congenital ZIKV infection is not yet known, all infants born to women with laboratory evidence of possible recent ZIKV infection during pregnancy should receive postnatal neuroimaging and ZIKV testing in addition to a comprehensive newborn physical exam and hearing screen. Identification and follow-up care of infants born to women with laboratory evidence of possible recent ZIKV infection during pregnancy and infants with possible congenital ZIKV infection can ensure that appropriate clinical services are available [118]. CDC analyzed data from 15 US jurisdictions conducting population-based surveillance for birth defects potentially related to ZIKV infection. Jurisdictions were stratified into the following three groups:

1) those with documented local transmission of ZIKV during 2016;
2) one or more cases of confirmed, symptomatic, travel-associated ZIKV disease reported to CDC per 100,000 residents; and

3) less than one case of confirmed, symptomatic, travel-associated ZIKV disease reported to CDC per 100,000 residents.

A total of 2,962 infants and fetuses (3.0 per 1,000 live births; 95% CI = 2.9-3.2) met the case definition. In areas with local transmission there was a non-statistically significant increase in total birth defects potentially related to ZIKV infection from 2.8 cases per 1,000 live births in the first half of 2016 to 3.0 cases in the second half ($p = 0.10$). However, when NTD and other early brain malformations were excluded, the prevalence of birth defects strongly linked to congenital ZIKV infection increased significantly, from 2.0 cases per 1,000 live births in the first half of 2016 to 2.4 cases in the second half, an increase of 29 more cases than expected ($p = 0.009$). These findings underscore the importance of surveillance for birth defects potentially related to ZIKV infection and the need for continued monitoring in areas at risk for zika [119]. Early identification of and intervention for neurodevelopmental problems can improve cognitive, social, and behavioral functioning. Pregnancies with laboratory evidence of confirmed or possible ZIKV infection and infants resulting from these pregnancies are included in the USZPIR and followed through active surveillance methods. An USZPIR report included data on children aged at least one year born in US territories and freely associated states. Receipt of reported follow-up care was assessed, and data were reviewed to identify zika-associated birth defects and neurodevelopmental abnormalities possibly associated with congenital ZIKV infection. Among 1,450 children of mothers with laboratory evidence of confirmed or possible ZIKV infection during pregnancy and with reported follow-up care, 76% had developmental screening or evaluation, 60% had postnatal neuroimaging, 48% had automated auditory brainstem response (ABR)-based hearing screen or evaluation, and 36% had an ophthalmological evaluation. Among evaluated children, 6% had at least one zika-associated birth defect identified, 9% had at least one neurodevelopmental abnormality possibly associated with congenital ZIKV infection identified, and 1% had both. One in seven evaluated children had a zika-associated birth defect, a neurodevelopmental abnormality possibly associated with congenital

ZIKV infection, or both reported to the USZPIR. Given that most children did not have evidence of all recommended evaluations, additional anomalies might not have been identified. Careful monitoring and evaluation of children born to mothers with evidence of ZIKV infection during pregnancy is essential for ensuring early detection of possible disabilities and early referral to intervention services [120]. In February 2016, CDC recommended:

1) routine testing for ZIKV infection of asymptomatic pregnant women living in areas with ongoing local ZIKV transmission at the first prenatal care visit;
2) re-testing during the second trimester for women who initially test negative; and
3) testing of pregnant women with signs or symptoms consistent with ZIKV disease (e.g., fever, rash, arthralgia, or conjunctivitis) at any time during pregnancy.

During January 1st, 2016-April 25th, 2017, US territories with local transmission of ZIKV reported 2,549 completed pregnancies (live births and pregnancy losses at any gestational age) with laboratory evidence of recent possible ZIKV infection; 5% of fetuses or infants resulting from these pregnancies had birth defects potentially associated with ZIKV infection. Among completed pregnancies with positive nucleic acid tests confirming zika infection identified in the first, second, and third trimesters, the percentage of fetuses or infants with possible zika-associated birth defects was 8%, 5%, and 4%, respectively. Among live-born infants, 59% had zika laboratory testing results reported to the pregnancy and infant registries. Identification and follow-up of infants born to women with laboratory evidence of recent possible ZIKV infection during pregnancy permits timely and appropriate clinical intervention services [121].

CDC has developed interim guidelines for health care providers in the US caring for pregnant women during a ZIKV outbreak. These guidelines include recommendations for pregnant women considering travel to an area with ZIKV transmission and recommendations for screening, testing, and management of pregnant returning travelers. Health care providers should ask all pregnant women about recent travel. Pregnant women with a history of travel to an area with ZIKV transmission and who report two or more symptoms consistent with ZIKV disease (acute onset of fever, maculopapular rash, arthralgia, or conjunctivitis) during or within two weeks of travel, or who have ultrasound findings of fetal microcephaly or intracranial calcifications, should be tested for ZIKV infection in consultation with their state or local health department. Testing is not indicated for women without a travel history to an area with ZIKV transmission. In pregnant women with laboratory evidence of ZIKV infection, serial ultrasound examination should be considered to monitor fetal growth and anatomy and referral to a maternal-fetal medicine or infectious disease specialist with expertise in pregnancy management is recommended [122]. Updated guidelines include a new recommendation to offer serological testing to asymptomatic pregnant women (women who do not report clinical illness consistent with ZIKV disease) who have traveled to areas with ongoing ZIKV transmission. Testing can be offered two to 12 weeks after pregnant women return from travel. This update also expands guidance to women who reside in areas with ongoing ZIKV transmission, and includes recommendations for screening, testing, and management of pregnant women and recommendations for counseling women of reproductive age (15-44 years). Pregnant women who reside in areas with ongoing ZIKV transmission have an ongoing risk for infection throughout their pregnancy. For pregnant women with clinical illness consistent with ZIKV disease, testing is recommended during the first week of illness. For asymptomatic pregnant women residing in areas with ongoing ZIKV transmission, testing is recommended at the initiation of prenatal care with mid-second trimester follow-up testing. Local health officials should determine when to implement testing of asymptomatic pregnant women based on information about levels of ZIKV transmission and laboratory capacity. Health care providers should discuss reproductive life plans, including pregnancy intention and timing, with women of reproductive age in the context of the potential risks associated with ZIKV infection [123].

CDC has updated its interim guidance for US health care providers caring for women of reproductive age with possible ZIKV exposure to include recommendations on counseling women and men with possible ZIKV exposure who are interested in conceiving. This guidance is based on limited available data on persistence of ZIKV RNA in blood and semen. Women who have ZIKV disease should wait at least eight weeks after symptom onset to attempt conception, and men with ZIKV disease should wait at least six months after symptom onset to attempt conception. Women and men with possible exposure to ZIKV but without clinical illness consistent with ZIKV disease should wait at least eight weeks after exposure to attempt conception. Possible exposure to ZIKV is defined as travel to or residence in an area of active ZIKV transmission, or sex (vaginal intercourse, anal intercourse, or fellatio) without a condom with a man who traveled to or resided in an area of active transmission. Women and men who reside in areas of active ZIKV transmission should talk with their health care provider about attempting conception [124]. CDC has updated its interim guidance for US health care providers caring for pregnant women with possible ZIKV exposure, to include the emerging data indicating that ZIKV RNA can be detected for prolonged periods in some pregnant women. To increase the proportion of pregnant women with ZIKV infection who receive a definitive diagnosis, CDC recommends expanding real-time RT-PCR testing. Possible exposures to ZIKV include travel to or residence in an area with active ZIKV transmission, or sex with a partner who has traveled to or resides in an area with active ZIKV transmission without using condoms or other barrier methods to prevent infection. Testing recommendations for pregnant women with possible ZIKV exposure who report clinical illness consistent with ZIKV disease (symptomatic pregnant women) are the same, regardless of their level of exposure (i.e., women with ongoing risk for possible exposure, including residence in or frequent travel to an area with active ZIKV transmission, as well as women living in areas without ZIKV transmission who travel to an area with active ZIKV transmission, or have unprotected sex with a partner who traveled to or resides in an area with active ZIKV transmission). Symptomatic pregnant women who are evaluated earlier than two weeks after symptom onset should receive serum and urine ZIKV RT-PCR testing. Symptomatic pregnant women who are evaluated two to 12 weeks after symptom onset should first receive a ZIKV IgM antibody test; if the IgM antibody test result is positive or equivocal, serum and urine RT-PCR testing should be performed. Testing recommendations for pregnant women with possible ZIKV exposure who do not report clinical illness consistent with ZIKV disease (asymptomatic pregnant women) differ based on the circumstances of possible exposure. For asymptomatic pregnant women who live in areas without active ZIKV transmission and who are evaluated earlier than two weeks after last possible exposure, RT-PCR testing should be performed. If the RT-PCR result is negative, a ZIKV IgM antibody test should be performed two to 12 weeks after the exposure. Asymptomatic pregnant women who do not live in an area with active ZIKV transmission, who are first evaluated two to 12 weeks after their last possible exposure should first receive a ZIKV IgM antibody test; if the IgM antibody test result is positive or equivocal, serum and urine RT-PCR should be performed. Asymptomatic pregnant women with ongoing risk for exposure to ZIKV should receive ZIKV IgM antibody testing as part of routine obstetric care during the first and second trimesters; immediate RT-PCR testing should be performed when IgM antibody test results are positive or equivocal [125]. CDC has updated the interim guidance for US health care providers caring for pregnant women with possible ZIKV exposure in response to:

1) declining prevalence of ZIKV disease in the WHO's Region of the Americas; and
2) emerging evidence indicating prolonged detection of ZIKV IgM antibodies.

ZIKV cases were first reported in the Americas during 2015-2016; however, the incidence of ZIKV disease has since declined. As the prevalence of ZIKV disease declines, the likelihood of false-positive test results increases. In addition, emerging epidemiological and laboratory data indicate that, as is the case with other Flaviviruses, ZIKV IgM antibodies can persist beyond 12 weeks after infection. Therefore, IgM test results cannot always reliably distinguish between an infection that occurred during the current pregnancy and one that occurred before the current pregnancy, particularly for women with possible ZIKV exposure before the current pregnancy. These limitations should be considered when counseling pregnant women about the risks and benefits of testing for ZIKV infection during pregnancy. This updated guidance emphasizes a shared decision-making model for testing and screening pregnant women, one in which patients and providers work together to make decisions about testing and care plans based on patient preferences and values, clinical judgment, and a balanced assessment of risks and expected outcomes [126].

Pregnant women in ZIKV-affected areas should protect themselves from mosquito bites by using air conditioning, screens, or nets when indoors, wearing long sleeves and pants, using permethrin-treated clothing and gear, and using insect repellents when outdoors. Pregnant and lactating women can use all US EPA-registered insect repellents according to the product label [127]. After reports of microcephaly and other adverse pregnancy outcomes in infants of mothers infected with ZIKV during pregnancy, CDC issued a travel alert on January 15th, 2016, advising pregnant women to consider postponing travel to areas with active transmission of ZIKV. On January 19th, CDC released interim guidelines for US health care providers caring for pregnant women with travel to an affected area, and an update was released on February 5th. As of February 17th, CDC had received reports of nine pregnant travelers with laboratory-confirmed ZIKV disease; 10 additional reports of ZIKV disease among pregnant women were under investigation. No ZIKV-related hospitalizations or deaths among pregnant women were reported. Pregnancy outcomes among the nine confirmed cases included two early pregnancy losses, two elective terminations, and three live births (two apparently healthy infants and one infant with severe microcephaly); two pregnancies (approximately 18 weeks' and 34 weeks' gestation) were continuing without known complications. Confirmed cases of ZIKV infection were reported among women who had traveled to one or more of the following nine areas with ongoing local transmission of ZIKV: American Samoa, Brazil, El Salvador, Guatemala, Haiti, Honduras, Mexico, Puerto Rico, and Samoa. US health care providers caring for pregnant women with possible ZIKV exposure during pregnancy should follow CDC guidelines for patient evaluation and management. ZIKV disease is a nationally notifiable condition [128]. Guidelines for US health care providers caring for infants born to mothers who traveled to or resided in areas with ZIKV transmission during pregnancy and guidelines to include infants and children with possible acute ZIKV disease contain a recommendation for routine care for infants born to mothers who traveled to or resided in areas with ZIKV transmission during pregnancy but did not receive ZIKV testing, when the infant has a normal head circumference, normal prenatal and postnatal ultrasounds (if performed), and normal physical examination. Acute ZIKV disease should be suspected in an infant or child aged <18 years who:

1) traveled to or resided in an affected area within the past two weeks; and
2) has at least two of the following manifestations: fever, rash, conjunctivitis, or arthralgia.

Since maternal-infant transmission of ZIKV during delivery is possible, acute ZIKV disease should also be suspected in an infant during the first two weeks of life:

1) whose mother traveled to or resided in an affected area within two weeks of delivery; and
2) who has at least two of the following manifestations: fever, rash, conjunctivitis, or arthralgia.

Evidence suggests that ZIKV illness in children is usually mild. As an arboviral disease, ZIKV disease is nationally notifiable. Health care providers should report suspected cases of ZIKV disease to their local, state, or territorial health departments to arrange testing and so that action can be taken to reduce the risk for local ZIKV transmission [129]. Laboratory testing is recommended for:

1) infants born to mothers with laboratory evidence of ZIKV infection during pregnancy; and
2) infants who have abnormal clinical or neuroimaging findings suggestive of CZS and a maternal epidemiological link suggesting possible transmission, regardless of maternal ZIKV test results.

Recommended infant laboratory evaluation includes both molecular (real-time RT-PCR) and serological (IgM) testing. Initial samples should be collected directly from the infant in the first two days of life, if possible; testing of cord blood is not recommended. A positive infant serum or urine RT-PCR test result confirms congenital ZIKV infection. Positive ZIKV IgM testing, with a negative RT-PCR result, indicates probable congenital ZIKV infection. In addition to infant ZIKV testing, initial evaluation of all infants born to mothers with laboratory evidence of ZIKV infection during pregnancy should include a comprehensive physical examination, including a neurological examination, postnatal head ultrasound, and standard newborn hearing screen. Infants with laboratory evidence of congenital ZIKV infection should have a comprehensive ophthalmological exam and hearing assessment by ABR testing before one month of age. Recommendations for follow-up of infants with laboratory evidence of congenital ZIKV infection depend on whether abnormalities consistent with CZS are present. Infants with abnormalities consistent with CZS should have a coordinated evaluation by multiple specialists within the first month of life; additional evaluations will be needed within the first year of life, including assessments of vision, hearing, feeding, growth, and neurodevelopmental and endocrine function. Families and caregivers will also need ongoing psycho-social support and assistance with coordination of care. Infants with laboratory evidence of congenital ZIKV infection without apparent abnormalities should have ongoing developmental monitoring and screening by the primary care provider; repeat hearing testing is recommended [130]. However, there are few published reports describing postnatally acquired ZIKV disease among children. During January 2015-July 2016, a total of 158 cases of confirmed or probable postnatally acquired ZIKV disease among children aged <18 years were reported to CDC from US. The median age was 14 years (range = one month to 17 years), and 88 (56%) were female. Two (1%) patients were hospitalized; none developed GBS, and none died. All reported cases were travel-associated. Overall, 129 (82%) children had rash, 87 (55%) had fever, 45 (29%) had conjunctivitis, and 44 (28%) had arthralgia. Health care providers should consider a diagnosis of ZIKV disease in children who have an epidemiological risk factor and clinically compatible illness, and should report cases to their state or local health department [131]. It is critical that pediatricians understand its epidemiology, clinical presentation, clinical sequelae, and management. The field of clinical research in ZIKV has rapidly evolved over recent months. It is critical that pediatricians continue to stay up-to-date with the continuously evolving understanding of the clinical aspects of ZIKV to ensure optimal identification and management of affected infants and children. Given the recent changes in CDC guidelines to limit screening of asymptomatic pregnant women in the US with possible ZIKV exposure, comprehensive ZIKV clinical knowledge becomes even more crucial [132-134].

In the past six years, ZIKV has emerged from obscurity onto the world stage-traversing and transcending clinical specialties, basic science disciplines, and public health efforts. Due to the fact that ZIKV can be sexually transmitted, there is a potential risk for disease transmission at several stages of assisted reproduction. Such a possibility poses a serious challenge to couples pursing fertility with assisted reproductive technologies (ART). ZIKV can be transmitted from infected men and women through vaginal, oral, or anal intercourse. ZIKV RNA has been detected in blood, semen, cervical mucus, and vaginal fluid. Currently, the CDC recommends that infected men wait six months, and infected women eight weeks, prior to attempting pregnancy. Reproductive tissue donors should wait six months before giving a specimen. Further study of ZIKV transmission in different reproductive tissues and establishment of validated testing methods for viral disease transmissibility are urgently needed. Reproductive technologists need to establish screening, testing, and laboratory protocols aimed to reduce the risk of ZIKV transmission during assisted reproduction [135]. Indeed, the spread of ZIKV has serious implications for the specialty of reproductive endocrinology and infertility. Patients, practices, and labs – worldwide and specifically in the US – have been impacted by this teratogenic, sexually transmitted, largely asymptomatic virus. While the WHO's PHEIC designation has lapsed as major epidemics have subsided and understanding of risks is in part clarified, the acute and long-term threat to pregnant patients is not over. The risk of wider spread in the US is not insignificant, the subtler and long-ranging consequences beyond microcephaly are not fully known, large geographic areas of risk still contain naïve populations, and whether zika will continue to be an intermittent risk in endemic areas is uncertain. Staying up to date with the burgeoning research on ZIKV is an important objective for all health care providers [136-138].

Given the extensive and variable fetal and newborn presentations/ complications associated with prenatal ZIKV infection, and the dearth of information provided, knowledge gaps are evident. Studies on this matter involve both rare outcomes and rare exposures and methodological choices are not straightforward. Cohort studies will surely offer more robust evidences, but their efficiency must be enhanced. A study can be statistically more efficient than another if its estimates are more accurate (precise and valid), even if the studies involve the same number of subjects. Sample size and specific design strategies can enhance or impair the statistical efficiency of a study, depending on how the subjects are distributed in subgroups pertinent to the analysis. In most ZIKV during pregnancy cohort studies to date there is an *a priori* identification of the source population (pregnant women, regardless of their exposure status) which is then sampled or included in its entirety (census). Subsequently, the group of pregnant women is classified according to exposure (presence or absence of ZIKV during pregnancy), respecting the exposed/unexposed ratio in the source population. The sample selection can be done from the *a priori* identification of groups of pregnant women exposed and unexposed to ZIKV during pregnancy. This method will allow for an oversampling (even 100%) of pregnant women with ZKV during pregnancy and an optimized sampling from the general population of pregnant women unexposed to ZIKV during pregnancy, saving resources in the unexposed group and improving the expected number of incident cases (outcomes) overall [139]. Mathematical modeling analysis using reported outcome data suggests that surveillance for these outcomes should begin as soon as an outbreak is detected and should continue for 40 weeks after the outbreak ends [140]. A non-human primate (NHP) model of congenital ZIKV infection can help fill the gaps in knowledge where tissue studies are required to define viral pathogenesis and identify targets for therapeutic intervention. This model system has already identified critical features of ZIKV pathogenesis in congenital infection. Before translating these NHP studies to human clinical trials, we must understand the similarities and differences between human and NHP fetal immune system development, neural development, and infant assessment tools. Because of the overall similarity between fetal and infant development in humans and NHP, this NHP model can complement human clinical trials by defining immune correlates of protection and evaluating therapeutic interventions [141]. Further research and comprehensive reporting may provide a better understanding of ZIKV infection in pregnancy and attendant maternal/fetal complications. This knowledge could inform the creation of effective and evidence-based strategies, guidelines, and recommendations aimed at the management of maternal ZIKV infection. Adherence to current best practice guidelines for prenatal care among health providers is encouraged in the context of maternal ZIKV infection [142-148].

DIAGNOSIS

Diagnosis of ZIKV infection should be suspected in individuals with the appropriate symptomatology and exposure history. Diagnostic tests are available and vary based on symptom duration [149]. Diagnostic testing for ZIKV infection can be accomplished using both molecular and serological methods. For persons with suspected ZIKV disease, a positive real-time RT-PCR result confirms ZIKV infection, but a negative RT-PCR result does not exclude infection. In these cases, IgM and neutralizing antibody testing can identify additional recent ZIKV infections. However, ZIKV antibody test results can be difficult to interpret because of cross-reactivity with other Flaviviruses, which can preclude identification of the specific infecting virus, especially when the person previously was infected with or vaccinated against a related Flavivirus. This is important because the results of ZIKV and DENV testing will guide clinical management. Pregnant women with laboratory evidence of ZIKV infection should be evaluated and managed for possible adverse pregnancy outcomes and be reported to the USZPIR or the Puerto Rico ZAPSS for clinical follow-up. All patients with clinically suspected dengue should have proper management to reduce the risk for hemorrhage and shock. If serological testing indicates recent Flavivirus infection that could be caused by either ZIKV or DENV, patients should be clinically managed for both infections because they might have been infected with either virus [150]. A confirmed case of ZIKV infection is defined as a positive result for ZIKV testing by RT-PCR for ZIKV in a blood or urine specimen. A presumptive case is defined as a positive result by ZIKV IgM ELISA and a negative result by DENV IgM ELISA, or a positive test result by ZIKV IgM ELISA in a pregnant woman. An unspecified Flavivirus case is defined as positive or equivocal results for both ZIKV and DENV by IgM ELISA [151-155].

The RNA of the ZIKV has been identified in samples of brain tissue, placenta, and amniotic fluid of children with microcephaly and in the still-born infants of women infected by zika during pregnancy. The RT-PCR test is recommended to detect viral RNA, and serological tests (IgM ELISA and neutralizing antibodies) should be conducted to confirm infection by zika. The differential diagnosis includes infection by DENV and CHIKV [156]. Urine and saliva have been previously established as useful tools in ZIKV diagnosis. The detection of infectious ZIKV particles in urine and saliva of patients during the acute phase may represent a critical factor in the spread of the virus. The epidemiological relevance of this finding, regarding the contribution of alternative non-vectorial ZIKV transmission routes, needs further investigation [157]. Rhesus macaques are susceptible to infection by an Asian-lineage ZIKV closely related to strains currently circulating in the Americas. Following subcutaneous inoculation, ZIKV RNA is detected in plasma one day post infection (d.p.i.) in all animals, and is also present in saliva, urine, and CSF. Non-pregnant and pregnant animals remain viremic for 21 days and for up to at least 57 days, respectively. Neutralizing antibodies are detected by 21 d.p.i. Re-challenge 10 weeks after the initial challenge results in no detectable virus replication, indicating protective immunity against homologous strains. Therefore, Asian-lineage ZIKV infection of Rhesus macaques provides a relevant animal model for studying pathogenesis and evaluating potential interventions against human infection, including during pregnancy [158-160].

CDC has developed interim guidelines for health care providers in the US who are caring for infants born to mothers who traveled to or resided in an area with ZIKV transmission during pregnancy. These guidelines include recommendations for the testing and management of these infants. Pediatric health care providers should work closely with obstetric providers to identify infants whose mothers were potentially infected with ZIKV during pregnancy (based on travel to or residence in an area with ZIKV transmission), and review fetal ultrasounds and maternal testing for ZIKV infection. ZIKV testing is recommended for:

1) infants with microcephaly or intracranial calcifications born to women who traveled to or resided in an area with ZIKV transmission while pregnant; or
2) infants born to mothers with positive or inconclusive test results for ZIKV infection.

For infants with laboratory evidence of a possible congenital ZIKV infection, additional clinical evaluation and follow-up is recommended. Health care providers should contact their state or territorial health department to facilitate testing [161]. CDC has updated its interim guidance for US health care providers caring for infants with possible congenital ZIKV infection in response to recently published updated guidance for health care providers caring for pregnant women with possible ZIKV exposure, unknown sensitivity and specificity of currently available diagnostic tests for congenital ZIKV infection, and recognition of additional clinical findings associated with congenital ZIKV infection. All infants born to mothers with possible ZIKV exposure during pregnancy should receive a standard evaluation at birth and at each subsequent well-child visit including a comprehensive physical examination, age-appropriate vision screening and developmental monitoring and screening using validated tools, and newborn hearing screen at birth, preferably using ABR methodology. Specific guidance for laboratory testing and clinical evaluation are provided for three clinical scenarios in the setting of possible maternal ZIKV exposure:

1) infants with clinical findings consistent with CZS regardless of maternal testing results;
2) infants without clinical findings consistent with CZS who were born to mothers with laboratory evidence of possible ZIKV infection; and
3) infants without clinical findings consistent with CZS who were born to mothers without laboratory evidence of possible ZIKV infection.

Infants in the first two scenarios should receive further testing and evaluation for ZIKV, whereas for the third group, further testing and clinical evaluation for ZIKV are not recommended. Health care providers should remain alert for abnormal findings (e.g., postnatal-onset microcephaly and eye abnormalities without microcephaly) in infants with possible congenital ZIKV exposure without apparent abnormalities at birth [162].

The rapid spread of ZIKV across the WHO's Region of the Americas has had a direct effect on the US health care delivery system. CDC recommends ZIKV testing for potentially exposed persons with signs or symptoms consistent with ZIKV disease, and recommends that health care providers offer testing to asymptomatic pregnant women within 12 weeks of exposure. During January 3rd-March 5th, 2016, ZIKV testing was performed for 4,534 persons who traveled to or moved from areas with active ZIKV transmission; 3,335 (73.6%) were pregnant women. Among persons who received testing, 1,541 (34.0%) reported at least one ZIKV-associated sign or symptom (e.g., fever, rash, arthralgia, or conjunctivitis), 436 (9.6%) reported at least one other clinical sign or symptom only, and 2,557 (56.4%) reported no signs or symptoms. Among 1,541 persons with one or more ZIKV-associated symptoms who received testing, 182 (11.8%) had confirmed ZIKV infection. Among the 2,557 asymptomatic persons who received testing, 2,425 (94.8%) were pregnant women, seven (0.3%) of whom had confirmed ZIKV infection. Although risk for ZIKV infection might vary based on exposure-related factors (e.g., location and duration of travel), in the current setting in US, where there is no local transmission, most asymptomatic pregnant women who receive testing do not have ZIKV infection [163]. Hospitals in NYC have been implementing prevention and response efforts consistent with CDC guidance. As of September 21st, 2016, a total of 715 cases of laboratory-confirmed ZIKV disease had been diagnosed in New York state among travelers who returned from affected areas, their sexual contacts, or infants infected in utero. This represents the highest number of reported cases in any state to date, and underscores the importance of health care systems preparing to care for patients with possible ZIKV disease. Building upon a framework that was established in 2014 to screen patients for possible exposure to EBOV disease, NYC Health Hospitals, the largest municipal health care delivery system in the US, implemented a Zika Preparedness and Response Action Plan (Zika Action Plan) to address the threat from zika and ensure appropriate patient care. The plan developed by NYC Health Hospitals includes universal travel screening, signage depicting areas with active ZIKV transmission, clinical and epidemiological evaluation for possible ZIKV exposure, diagnostic testing for ZIKV infection and linking of infected patients to appropriate specialists, and education on ZIKV disease and preventive measures (e.g., avoiding travel to areas with active ZIKV transmission) [164]. The first patients with laboratory-confirmed cases of ZIKV disease in American Samoa had symptom onset in January 2016. In response, the ASDoH implemented mosquito control measures, strategies to protect pregnant women, syndromic surveillance based on electronic health record (EHR) reports, ZIKV testing of persons with one or more signs or symptoms of ZIKV disease (fever, rash, arthralgia, or conjunctivitis), and routine testing of all asymptomatic pregnant women in accordance with CDC guidance. All collected blood and urine specimens were shipped to the Hawaii Department of Health Laboratory for ZIKV testing and to CDC for confirmatory testing. Early in the response, collection and testing of specimens from pregnant women was prioritized over the collection from symptomatic non-pregnant patients because of limited testing and shipping capacity. The weekly numbers of suspected ZIKV disease cases declined from an average of six per week in January-February 2016 to one per week in May 2016. By August, the EHR-based syndromic surveillance indicated a return to pre-outbreak levels. The last ZIKV disease case detected by real-time RT-PCR occurred in a patient who had symptom onset on June 19th, 2016. In August 2016, ASDoH requested CDC support in assessing whether local transmission had been reduced or interrupted and in proposing a timeline for discontinuation of routine testing of asymptomatic pregnant women. An end date (October 15th, 2016) was determined for active mosquito-borne transmission of ZIKV and a timeline was developed for discontinuation of routine screening of asymptomatic pregnant women in American Samoa (conception after December 10th, 2016, with permissive testing for asymptomatic women who conceived through April 15th, 2017) [165].

The detection of suspected cases by the surveillance system depends on the case definition adopted. As the laboratory diagnosis of zika infection still relies on the use of expensive and complex molecular techniques with low sensitivity due to a narrow window of detection, most suspected cases are not confirmed by laboratory tests, mainly reserved for pregnant women and newborns. In this context, an accurate definition of a suspected zika case is crucial in order for the surveillance system to gauge the magnitude of an epidemic. In areas where multiple arboviruses circulate, the presence of rash with pruritus or conjunctival hyperemia, without any other general clinical manifestations such as fever, petechia, or anorexia is the best zika case definition [166]. The identify-isolate-inform (3I) tool, originally conceived for initial detection and management of EBOV disease patients in the emergency department, and later adjusted for measles and Middle East Respiratory Syndrome (MERS), can be adapted for real-time use for any emerging infectious disease. Following an assessment of epidemiological risk, including travel to countries with mosquitoes that transmit ZIKV, patients are further investigated if clinically indicated. If after a rapid evaluation, zika or other arthropod-borne diseases are the only concern, isolation (contact, droplet, and airborne) is unnecessary. The modified 3I tool can facilitate rapid analysis and triggering of appropriate actions for patients presenting to the emergency department at risk for zika [167]. Determining the viral cause of a rash presents significant diagnostic challenges. ZIKV has re-emerged in the Pacific with local transmission from imported cases. Climate change, global warming, and spillover of zoonotic viruses are contributing to the emergence and spread of viral diseases. Important clues to the diagnosis of viral exanthems include their distribution and morphology, geographic location, and potential exposure to vector-borne or blood-borne viruses. Diagnosis is commonly made via serology, nucleic acid tests or, rarely, viral culture. Skin biopsy is not usually required [168]. Defining the tissue pathology associated with the various disease manifestations provides insight into pathogenesis and diagnosis, and potentially future prevention and treatment, of ZIKV infections. Pathological findings associated with ZIKV infection are characteristic but not specific. In CZS, tissue pathology is due to direct viral infection of neural structures, whereas in GBS, pathology is likely due to a post-viral, aberrant host-directed immune response. Both fetal and placental pathology specimens are useful for ZIKV diagnosis by molecular and immunohistochemical (IHC) assays; however, the implications of ZIKV detection in placentas from second- and third-trimester normal live births are unclear, as the potential postnatal effects of late gestational exposure remain to be seen [169]. Detection of ZIKV RNA in clinical and tissue specimens can provide definitive laboratory evidence of recent ZIKV infection. Whereas duration of viremia is typically short, prolonged detection of ZIKV RNA in placental, fetal, and neonatal brain tissue has been reported and can provide key diagnostic information by confirming recent ZIKV infection. In accordance with recent guidance, CDC provides ZIKV testing of placental and fetal tissues in clinical situations where this information could add diagnostic value. A report described the evaluation of formalin-fixed paraffin-embedded (FFPE) tissue specimens tested for ZIKV infection in 2016 and the contribution of this testing to the public health response. Among 546 live births with possible maternal ZIKV exposure, for which placental tissues were submitted by the 50 states and DC, 60 (11%) were positive by ZIKV RT-PCR. Among 81 pregnancy losses for which placental and/or fetal tissues were submitted, 18 (22%) were positive by ZIKV RT-PCR. ZIKV RT-PCR was positive on placental tissues from 38/363 (10%) live births with maternal serological evidence of recent unspecified Flavivirus infection and from 9/86 (10%) with negative maternal ZIKV IgM where possible maternal exposure occurred >12 weeks before serum collection. These results demonstrate that ZIKV RT-PCR testing of tissue specimens can provide a confirmed diagnosis of recent maternal ZIKV infection [170].

CZS is a recognizable pattern of structural anomalies and functional disabilities secondary to CNS and, perhaps, PNS damage. Although many of the components of this syndrome, such as cognitive, sensory, and motor disabilities, are shared by other congenital infections, there are five features that are rarely seen with other congenital infections or are unique to congenital ZIKV infection:

1) severe microcephaly with partially collapsed skull;
2) thin cerebral cortices with subcortical calcifications;
3) macular scarring and focal pigmentary retinal mottling;
4) congenital contractures; and
5) marked early hypertonia and symptoms of extrapyramidal involvement.

Although the full spectrum of adverse reproductive outcomes caused by ZIKV infection is not yet determined, a distinctive phenotype – the CZS

– has emerged. Recognition of this phenotype by clinicians for infants and children can help ensure appropriate etiological evaluation and comprehensive clinical investigation to define the range of anomalies in an affected infant as well as determine essential follow-up and ongoing care [171]. Neuropathological findings in CZS helped to understand its pathogenetic mechanisms. The most relevant post-mortem findings in the CNS of fetuses and neonates infected with ZIKV early in gestation are microcephaly with *ex vacuo* ventriculomegaly and large head circumference associated with obstructive hydrocephalus due to severe mid-brain and aqueduct distortion. Babies with severe brain lesions are born with arthrogryposis. Histologically, there is extensive destruction of the hemispheric parenchyma, calcifications, various disturbances of neuronal migration, reactive gliosis, microglial hyperplasia, and occasional perivascular cuffs of lymphocytes, also in the meninges. Hypoplastic lesions secondary to the lack of descending nerve fibers include small basis pontis, pyramids, and spinal corticospinal tracts. Cerebellar hypoplasia is also common. Severe nerve motor nerve cell loss is observed in the anterior horn of the spinal cord. A spectrum of neuropathological changes, from severe microcephaly to obstructive hydrocephalus, is observed. The severity of the lesions is directly related to the gestational age, the most severe occurring when the mother is infected in the first trimester. Infection of progenitor cells at the germinal matrix is demonstrated. The lack of spinal motor neurons is responsible for fetal akinesia and consequent arthrogryposis [172, 173].

In 1984, Chervenak et al. proposed criteria for the prenatal ultrasound diagnosis of microcephaly as at least three standard deviations (SD) from the mean. Despite improvements in medicine, these criteria have not been reevaluated in 30 years. The 1984 ultrasound criteria for microcephaly remain valid. Physicians today have two alternatives: either use the three-SD cutoff as recommended by Chervenak et al. and endorsed by the SMFM or develop a new dataset for one's population with statistical validation [174-176]. A wide range of clinical-radiological findings of congenital ZIKV infections were reported in the literature, such as microcephaly, overlapping sutures, cortical migrational and *corpus callosum* abnormalities, intracranial calcifications, ventriculomegaly, brain stem and cerebellar malformations, spinal cord involvement, and joint contractures. ZIKV is also related to other severe neurological manifestations in grown-up individuals such as GBS and encephalomyelitis [177]. The most frequently observed radiological findings are microcephaly and decreased brain parenchymal volume associated with lissencephaly, ventriculomegaly secondary to the lack of brain tissue (not hypertensive), and coarse and anarchic calcifications mainly involving the subcortical cortical transition, and the basal ganglia. Although it cannot be concluded that there is a definitive pathognomonic radiographic pattern of microcephaly caused by ZIKV, gross calcifications and anarchic distribution involving the subcortical cortical transition and the basal ganglia, in association with lissencephaly and in the absence of hypertensive ventriculomegaly, are characteristic of this type of infection [178]. Neuroimaging investigation contributes to the prenatal detection of microcephaly and other brain abnormalities in cases of intrauterine ZIKV infection. Neuroimaging is based antenatally on two-dimensional and three-dimensional ultrasound and fetal magnetic resonance imaging (MRI), whereas computed tomography (CT) scan is performed postnatally. Although neuropathology associated with intrauterine ZIKV infection is characterized by non-specific findings of brain disorder, reduced cortical gyration and white-matter hypomyelination or dysmyelination and cerebellar hypoplasia have been consistently observed in the majority of fetuses and newborns. Prenatal or postnatal genetic workup should be carried out to exclude cases of primary microcephaly. Follow-up should rely upon MRI and CT scan as well as neuropediatrician to better define developmental outcome in survivors [179-181].

Ethical and Social Issues

While until recently the small and isolated zika outbreaks in Eastern Asia and Pacific Islands had been overlooked, the large-scale outbreak that started in Brazil in 2015 and the increase of microcephaly cases in the same place and time made media headlines. Considered as harmless until recently, zika has given rise to an important global crisis that poses not only health challenges but also environmental, economic, social, and ethical challenges for states and people around the world [182]. In the first phases of an infectious outbreak, health authorities have to face the challenge of communicating uncertainty. Just when the attention of the public is at the top, information about what is going on is usually still missing. This is the case of zika crisis in Latin America, where an association with microcephaly in newborns and neurological complications have been described. Despite this, and even if the risk would be mainly limited to pregnant women, zika threat is perceived by the general public as greater than others, such as those from dengue or flu. Some peculiarities of this outbreak explain such a gap between real and perceived risk. Nevertheless, in such a situation, WHO and other health authorities have the duty to act out of an abundance of caution, aware of the lose-lose game they are going through: if they raise alarm, and this subsided, they could be accused to fuel people's fears because of economic interests, as it happened in 2009 A (H1N1) pandemic; if they underestimate the threat, they could find themselves in front of a global tragedy [183].

The zika pandemic provides biomedical scientists, clinicians, public health advocates, and governments a unique opportunity to advance reproductive justice. The circumstances in which pregnancies occur are morally relevant to women's reproductive life decisions, to the provision of reproductive health care, and to the development of reproductive health policy. Whether the zika pandemic might foster context-driven reproductive pandemic planning and response is yet to be determined. Maintaining the status quo will surely increase a range of global health disparities and further stratify reproduction, producing predictable and preventable outcomes in which some people receive the necessary care and resources to achieve family building while others are neglected. Women and men should be able to count on biomedical researchers to answer the questions that need answering without undue influence from political agendas. Women should be able to continue pregnancies and count on public health assistance and help for children with zika-related disabilities, or prevent or end a zika-affected pregnancy. Pandemic responses that don't further these ends are morally unacceptable [184]. Public health officials, policymakers, and international organizations are considering interventions to address health consequences of the zika epidemic. To date, public health responses have focused on mosquito vector eradication, sexual and reproductive health services, knowledge and technology including diagnostic test and vaccine development, and health system preparedness [185]. As ZIKV continues to spread, decisions regarding resource allocations to control the outbreak underscore the need for a tool to weigh policies according to their cost and the health burden they could avert. For example, to combat zika outbreak the US President requested the allocation of $ 1.8 billion from Congress in February 2016. The commitments and the proposal are likely to be cost-effective, whereas the cost-effectiveness of genetically modified mosquitoes depends on the country of implementation. Current estimates suggest that the health burden from microcephaly and GBS warrants substantial expenditures focused on ZIKV control. Results justify the funding committed in Costa Rica and Brazil and many aspects of the budget outlined in the US President's proposal. As data continue to be collected, new parameter estimates can be customized in real-time to provide updated estimates on cost-effectiveness of interventions and inform policy decisions in country-specific settings [186].

Much of the fear and uncertainty around zika epidemics stem from potential association between ZIKV complications on infected pregnant women and risk of their babies being born with microcephaly and other neurological abnormalities. However, much remains unknown about its mode of transmission, diagnosis, and long-term pathogenesis. Worries of these unknowns necessitate the need for effective and efficient psycho-social programs and medical-legal strategies to alleviate and mitigate ZIKV related burdens. In this light, local and global efforts in maintaining fundamental health principles of moral, medical and legal decision-making policies, and interventions to preserve and promote individual and collective Human Rights, autonomy, protection of the most vulnerable, equity, dignity, integrity, and beneficence that should not be confused and relegated by compassionate humanitarian assistance and support. Further long-term cross-borders operational research is required in elucidating zika-related population-based epidemiology, ethical-medical, and societal implications in guiding evidence-based local and global ZIKV maternal-child health complications related approaches and interventions. Meeting basic health needs (i.e., preventive measures), together with research and development conducive to a vaccine for global zika immunization program in most vulnerable and affected countries and worldwide or treatment for the ZIKV should be priorities [187]. Since a vaccine or anti-viral therapy is not yet available, current means of disease prevention involve protection from mosquito bites, excluding pregnant females from traveling to zika-endemic territories, and practicing safe sex in those countries. Importantly, in countries where zika is reported as endemic, caution is advised in planning to conceive a baby until such time as the apparent association between infection with the virus and microcephaly is either confirmed or refuted. The question arises as to what advice is appropriate to give in more economically developed countries distant to the current epidemic and in which zika has not yet been reported. Despite understandable concern among the general public that has been fueled by the media, in regions where zika is not present, such as North America, Europe, and Australia, at this time any outbreak (initiated by an infected traveler returning from an endemic area) would very probably be contained locally. Since *Aedes* spp. has very limited spatial dispersal, overlapping high population densities of mosquitoes and humans would be needed to sustain a focus of infection. However, as *A. aegypti* is distinctly anthropophilic, future control strategies for zika should be considered in tandem with the continuing threat to human well-being that is presented by dengue, yellow fever, and Japanese encephalitis, all of which are transmitted by the same vector species [188].

Zika's impact on infants may shift the terms of debate about abortion access [189]. The focus on abortion legalization in the aftermath of the zika outbreak is distracting for policy and lawmakers from what needs to be done to address the outbreak effectively [190]. The high number of cases in Brazil has been attributed to a failure of the state to contain the epidemic and protect the affected people, especially women. Therefore, the public health crisis created by zika exposed a stark conflict between Brazil's constitutional right to health and the long-standing violation of reproductive rights in the country. Although health is considered to be a right of all in Brazil, women struggle with barriers to reproductive services and lack of access to safe and legal abortions. In response to the epidemic, women's rights advocates have filed a lawsuit with Brazil's supreme court that requires the decriminalization of abortion upon the diagnosis of ZIKV. However, the selective decriminalization of abortion may lead to negative social consequences and further stigmatization of people with disabilities. A solution to the reproductive health crisis in Brazil must reconcile women's right to choose and the rights of people with disabilities [191].

The ZIKV epidemic and the possible devastating teratogenic effects of the virus represent a challenge. Health authorities have the responsibility to create programs that provide adequate preventive, medical, and psychological services to the affected population. The estimated risk of microcephaly in infants of mothers infected with ZIKV is 1% to 13% when the infection occurs in the first trimester of pregnancy. There is insufficient data to estimate the risk of microcephaly when infection occurs in the second or third trimester. Pregnant women and those in reproductive age are advised to avoid traveling to places where there is local transmission of the ZIKV. Human rights advocates have requested comprehensive sexual and reproductive health services that include expanded access to contraceptive methods including emergency contraception and safe abortion services. These strategies created a debate between the abortion rights and the right of the disabled. The discussion rests on the assumption that there are lives that are not worth living. Most people focus on the most severely affected patients, but few consider that the spectrum of disabilities associated with congenital zika infection is broad. The rights of children with disabilities and their dignity as individuals should be respected [192]. The uncertainty surrounding the possibility of congenital anomalies due to ZIKV infection during pregnancy bring a renewed debate about the rights of women to control their reproductive decisions. Current strategies, resources, and services aimed at prevention priorities fall short of responding to a clear framework regarding sexual reproductive health, rights, and justice. A comprehensive approach to reproduction, in times of zika, needs to empower women of reproductive age and their families to make decisions and to act on those decisions [193-195].

PREVENTION

As ZIKV continues to spread and further research is conducted regarding its teratogenic effects, the need for concise and effective education is critical to raise awareness, decrease the potential for maternal exposure, and reduce fetal risks. Therefore, the need for appropriate recognition, treatment, management, and prevention of the ZIKV disease prompts the necessity for further education and high-quality level research to be conducted and utilized [196]. Currently, no vaccine or medication exists to prevent or treat ZIKV infection. Persons residing in or traveling to areas of active ZIKV transmission should take steps to prevent ZIKV infection through prevention of mosquito bites [197]. Widespread ZIKV transmission in the Region of the Americas since 2015 has heightened the urgency of preparing for the possibility of expansion of mosquito-borne transmission of ZIKV during the mosquito seasons. CDC and other US government agencies have been working with state and local government partners on prevention and early detection of ZIKV infection and will increase these activities as part of their preparation for the anticipated emergence of mosquito-borne transmission of ZIKV in the continental US [198]. Health care providers must be equipped to provide appropriate advice to reproductive-aged patients for protection against the potentially devastating consequences of prenatal ZIKV exposure. All travelers should use personal protective measures against mosquito bites including insect repellents and protection of living areas against mosquito entry. Pregnant women should avoid travel to areas designated as being of concern because of ongoing ZIKV transmission. Women planning a pregnancy should consult with their health care provider and consider postponing travel to these areas. All other travelers may wish to consider deferring travel to designated areas based on risk tolerance, values, and preferences. In the absence of clear data, we make the assumption that viral shedding is unlikely to persist beyond six months for men and two months for non-pregnant women. Health care providers should take a travel history from their pregnant patients including relevant information related to the travel history of their partners. Screening and management recommendations are provided for all travelers including potentially contagious male partners, pregnant women (symptomatic and asymptomatic), and the fetus or infant of potentially infected women. Robust quantitative assessments for the full spectrum of ZIKV-associated risks are not possible. This reflects, among other things, uncertainties related to the likelihood of infection among travelers to ZIKV-affected areas, vertical transmission from mother to fetus, sexual transmission (from symptomatic or asymptomatic partners), and serious ZIKV-associated sequelae among travelers. Given this uncertainty, as well as the potentially severe effects of ZIKV infection on the fetus, recommendations are conservative [199].

Control measures include using insect repellents, aerial spraying of insecticides, eliminating mosquito breeding sites, covering water tanks, and using mosquito nets or door and window screens [200]. Reviews assessing the safety and toxicity of N,N-diethyl-meta-toluamide (DEET) conducted by the US EPA and the Canadian Pest Management Regulatory Agency (PMRA) conclude that DEET has low acute toxicity and does not appear to pose a significant health concern to humans when used as directed. Some experimental animal and limited epidemiological data suggest that prenatal pyrethroid (permethrin) exposure may adversely affect learning and behavior, but this level of evidence pales in comparison to the known risks of ZIKV to the fetal brain. The available evidence has led to the strong recommendation by the CDC for use of these products by pregnant women as personal protection against mosquito bites in the fight against ZIKV infection. This message has been affirmed by obstetrics and gynecology professional organizations. Because ZIKV is unlikely to be the last disease requiring vector control, those with environmental health expertise must continue to join with infectious disease specialists to communicate the potential vulnerability of the youngest (fetuses, infants, and young children) to vector-borne disease, both to the disease itself and to the strategies employed to mitigate the spread of such disease [201].

Outbreaks of mosquito-borne viral illnesses commonly occur after storms. As storms are predicted to worsen in intensity and frequency, mosquito-borne viruses, including the ZIKV are expected to spread, and with devastating consequences. An overlooked vector of the ZIKV, however, is men whose semen can transmit the virus at the time of sexual intercourse. Thus, although spread is primarily by *Aedes* spp. mosquitoes, instances of sexual transmission of ZIKV have been reported, and replicative virus has been isolated from semen of one man with hematospermia. On February 5th, 2016, CDC published recommendations for preventing sexual transmission of ZIKV. Updated prevention guidelines were published on February 23rd, with a further update on April 1st, 2016. During February 6th-22nd, 2016, CDC received reports of 14 instances of suspected sexual transmission of ZIKV. Among these, two laboratory-confirmed cases and four probable cases of ZIKV disease have been identified among women whose only known risk factor was sexual contact with a symptomatic male partner with recent travel to an area with ongoing ZIKV transmission. Two instances have been excluded based on additional information, and six others are still under investigation. State, territorial, and local public health departments, clinicians, and the public should be aware of current recommendations for preventing sexual transmission of ZIKV, particularly to pregnant women. Men who reside in or have traveled to an area of ongoing ZIKV transmission and have a pregnant partner should abstain from sexual activity or consistently and correctly use condoms during sex with their pregnant partner for the duration of the pregnancy [202]. The above recommendations apply to all men and women who have traveled to or reside in areas with active ZIKV transmission and their female or male sex partners. These recommendations are updated to include time intervals after travel to areas with active ZIKV transmission or after ZIKV infection for taking precautions to reduce the risk for sexual transmission. This guidance defines potential sexual exposure to ZIKV as any person who has had sex (i.e., vaginal intercourse, anal intercourse, or fellatio) without a condom with a man who has traveled to or resides in an area with active ZIKV transmission [203]. The recommendations are now updated to reduce the risk for sexual transmission of ZIKV from both men and women to their sex partners. This guidance defines potential sexual exposure to ZIKV as having had sex with a person who has traveled to or lives in an area with active ZIKV transmission when the sexual contact did not include a barrier to protect against infection. Such barriers include male or female condoms for vaginal or anal sex and other barriers for oral sex. Sexual exposure includes vaginal sex, anal sex, oral sex, or other activities that might expose a sex partner to genital secretions [204].

CDC has updated its interim guidance for persons with possible ZIKV exposure who are planning to conceive and interim guidance to prevent transmission of ZIKV through sexual contact, now combined into a single document. Possible ZIKV exposure is defined as travel to or residence in an area of active ZIKV transmission, or sex without a condom with a partner who traveled to or lived in an area of active transmission. Based on new though limited data, CDC now recommends that all men with possible ZIKV exposure who are considering attempting conception with their partner, regardless of symptom status, wait to conceive until at least six months after symptom onset (if symptomatic) or last possible ZIKV exposure (if asymptomatic). Recommendations for women planning to conceive remain unchanged: women with possible ZIKV exposure are recommended to wait to conceive until at least eight weeks after symptom onset (if symptomatic) or last possible ZIKV exposure (if asymptomatic). Couples with possible ZIKV exposure, who are not pregnant and do not plan to become pregnant, who want to minimize their risk for sexual transmission of ZIKV should use a condom or abstain from sex for the same periods for men and women described above. Women of reproductive age who have had or anticipate future ZIKV exposure who do not want to become pregnant should use the most effective contraceptive method that can be used correctly and consistently [205]. CDC has also updated the interim guidance for men with possible ZIKV exposure who:

1) are planning to conceive with their partner; or
2) want to prevent sexual transmission of ZIKV at any time.

CDC now recommends that men with possible ZIKV exposure who are planning to conceive with their partner wait for at least three months after symptom onset (if symptomatic) or their last possible ZIKV exposure (if asymptomatic) before engaging in unprotected sex. CDC now also recommends that for couples who are not trying to conceive, men can consider using condoms or abstaining from sex for at least three months after symptom onset (if symptomatic) or their last possible ZIKV exposure (if asymptomatic) to minimize their risk for sexual transmission of ZIKV. All other guidance for ZIKV remains unchanged. The definition of possible ZIKV exposure remains unchanged and includes travel to or residence in an area with risk for ZIKV transmission or sex without a condom with a partner who traveled to or lives in an area with risk for ZIKV transmission [206].

Current recommendations for preventing the sexual transmission of zika are inadequate and need to emphasize male reproductive responsibility, via expanding services for men's family planning and developing novel male contraceptives. To prevent the sexual transmission of zika, the WHO recommends that couples use condoms or abstain from sexual activity for at least six months when traveling in zika-infected areas. Strict adherence to these recommendations is neither practical nor adequate to address zika's sexual transmission. As up to 13% of couples who use condoms experience unintended pregnancy, semen and consequent viral exposure is imminent. The use of contraception beyond just barrier methods is essential. However, the burden of contraception largely falls upon women and efforts to prevent vertical transmission are often aimed at educating women, when the outcome is equally undesirable among their male partners. These short-comings highlight the lack of attention to men's options for family planning. Educating men about the full range of contraceptive options, correcting misconceptions about the efficacy of withdrawal and barrier contraceptive methods, increasing access to vasectomy, and developing novel male contraceptive options would allow shared responsibility for the prevention of unintended pregnancy and zika-related morbidity. Gaps in recommendations to prevent the sexual transmission of zika provide an opportunity to develop men's family planning initiatives and the range of accessible contraceptives to men [207]. Broad recommendations by government agencies and public health officials regarding avoidance of pregnancy for women at risk of acquiring ZIKV have theoretical and documented implications for abortion and contraception demand and access. Additional research is needed to better understand the impact of ZIKV health recommendations and advisories on women's decision making around pregnancy, as well as their impact on demand, access, and safety of family planning services [208, 209].

Because of the potential risks associated with ZIKV infection during pregnancy, CDC has recommended that health care providers discuss prevention of unintended pregnancy with women and couples who reside in areas of active ZIKV transmission and do not want to become pregnant. However, limitations in access to contraception in some of these areas might affect the ability to prevent an unintended pregnancy. In fact, in all these countries a large proportion of babies are still born out of unplanned pregnancies. Public health messaging on zika prevention has predominantly targeted women who know they are pregnant or intend to become pregnant, but not teenage females for whom unintended pregnancy is more likely. Vulnerabilities among this population to reproductive risks associated with zika are further amplified by restrictive abortion laws in several zika-impacted states. Key to prevention is enhanced, targeted public health messaging centered on teens nationally and particularly in certain high-risk regions [210]. Teenage girls are particularly at high risk, as they often lack access to preventive contraception methods, or the knowledge to use them appropriately. Nearly 20% of children born in Brazil today (~560,000 live births) are by teenage mothers. Birth incidence is far higher in the tropical and poorer northern states. However, in absolute terms most births occur in the populous southeastern states, matching to a large extent the geographic distribution of dengue (an indicator of suitable climatic and sociodemographic conditions for the circulation of *Aedes* mosquitoes). These findings indicate that recommendation to delay pregnancy will leave over half a million pregnant adolescents in Brazil vulnerable to infection every year if not accompanied by effective education and real access to prevention [211]. Individual health care providers may encounter health system barriers to providing evidence-based care. In Mexico, states with the highest unmet need for contraception are low-lying coastal states. The government recently announced an investment to combat zika but made no mention of family planning initiatives to assist women in preventing pregnancy. In Texas, the DSHS has issued recommendations to help women and men avoid mosquito bites; the issue of whether women should plan or avoid pregnancy is not addressed. Puerto Rico has the largest number of confirmed cases of ZIKV in the US and territories. Recently, the CDC Foundation launched the Zika Contraception Access Network (Z-CAN), which provides contraceptives at no cost to participating clinics in Puerto Rico. ZIKV highlights weaknesses in health systems that make it difficult for women to use contraception if they want to delay births. Women across the globe, with or without ZIKV, need access to contraception to prevent unintended pregnancy, and health care providers require functioning health systems that offer support to ensure access is a reality [212].

In response to the ZIKV threat, the WHO is strategically targeting prevention of infection in pregnant women and funding contraception in epidemic regions. The damaging effects of ZIKV can be reduced using a seasonal window of opportunity for conception that may minimize maternal exposure. Like other acute viral infections – including the related Flavivirus, DENV – the transmission of ZIKV is anticipated to be seasonal. By seasonally planning pregnancy, this aspect of pathogen ecology can be leveraged to align sensitive periods of gestation with the low-transmission season [213]. However, the effectiveness of this policy in reducing prenatal ZIKV infection has yet to be quantified. With 50% adherence to recommendations to delay pregnancy by nine to 24 months, the cumulative incidence of prenatal ZIKV infections is likely to decrease by 17% to 44%, whereas recommendations to delay pregnancy by six or fewer months are likely to increase prenatal infections by 2% to 7%. This paradoxical exacerbation of prenatal ZIKV exposure is due to an elevated risk for pregnancies to shift toward the peak of the outbreak. Pregnancy delays can have a substantial effect on reducing cases of microcephaly but risks exacerbating the ZIKV outbreak if the duration is not sufficient. Duration of the delay, population adherence, and the timing of initiation of the intervention must be carefully considered [214].

ZIKV infection during pregnancy remains a serious health threat in Puerto Rico. As of March 16th, 2016, the highest number of ZIKV disease cases in the US and territories were reported from Puerto Rico. The number of cases will likely rise with increasing mosquito activity in affected areas, resulting in increased risk for transmission to pregnant women. High rates of unintended and adolescent pregnancies in Puerto Rico suggest that, in the context of this outbreak, access to contraception might need to be improved. CDC estimates that 138,000 women of reproductive age (aged 15-44 years) in Puerto Rico do not desire pregnancy and are not using one of the most effective or moderately effective contraceptive methods, and therefore might experience an unintended pregnancy. CDC and other federal and local partners are seeking to expand access to contraception for these persons. Such efforts have the potential to increase contraceptive access and use, reduce unintended pregnancies, and lead to fewer adverse pregnancy and birth outcomes associated with ZIKV infection during pregnancy. The assessment of challenges and resources related to contraceptive access in Puerto Rico might be a useful model for other areas with active transmission of ZIKV [215]. From January 1st, 2016 through March 29th, 2017, Puerto Rico reported approximately 3,300 pregnant women with laboratory evidence of possible ZIKV infection. There is currently no vaccine or intervention to prevent the adverse effects of ZIKV infection during pregnancy; therefore, prevention has been the focus of public health activities, especially for pregnant women. CDC and the PRDH analyzed data from the Pregnancy Risk Assessment Monitoring System – Zika Postpartum Emergency Response (PRAMS-ZPER) survey conducted from August through December 2016 among Puerto Rico residents with a live birth. Most women (98.1%) reported using at least one measure to avoid mosquitoes in their home environment. However, only 45.8% of women reported wearing mosquito repellent daily, and 11.5% reported wearing pants and shirts with long sleeves daily. Approximately one third (38.5%) reported abstaining from sex or using condoms consistently throughout pregnancy. Overall, 76.9% of women reported having been tested for ZIKV by their health care provider during the first or second trimester of pregnancy. These results can be used to assess and refine ZIKV infection prevention messaging and interventions for pregnant women and to reinforce measures to promote prenatal testing for zika [216]. As of May 2nd, 2017, the USVI, comprising St. Thomas, St. John, and St. Croix, had reported 1,021 probable or confirmed cases of ZIKV disease in its population of approximately 100,000; 222 symptomatic and asymptomatic pregnant women in the USVI had tested positive for ZIKV. In January 2016, USVI Department of Health (DOH) initiated zika response measures, including surveillance, vector control, and a communications program. Interventions included education and outreach, distribution of zika prevention kits to pregnant women in the USVI, and provision of free ZIKV laboratory testing and vector control services. In November 2016, USVI DOH staff members conducted interviews with convenience samples of community members and pregnant women to gather feedback about current and proposed interventions. Pregnant women reported taking a median of two actions to protect themselves from zika, with repellent use being the most commonly reported action. Community members reported taking a median of one action and were supportive of several proposed vector control approaches. Whereas multiple pregnant women and community members reported hearing messages about the cause and consequences of ZIKV infections, few recalled messages about specific actions they could take to protect themselves. Integrating evaluation into response measures permits ongoing assessment of intervention effectiveness and supports improvement to serve the population's needs [217].

CDC prevention efforts include mosquito surveillance and control, targeted education about ZIKV and condom use to prevent sexual transmission, and guidance for providers on contraceptive counseling to reduce unintended pregnancy. To estimate the prevalence of contraceptive use among non-pregnant and postpartum women at risk for unintended pregnancy and sexually active female high school students living in the 41 states where mosquito-borne transmission might be possible, CDC used 2011-2013 and 2015 survey data from four state-based surveillance systems: the Behavioral Risk Factor Surveillance System (BRFSS, 2011-2013), which surveys adult women; the PRAMS (2013) and the Maternal and Infant Health Assessment (MIHA, 2013), which surveys women with a recent live birth; and the Youth Risk Behavior Survey (YRBS, 2015), which surveys students in grades nine to 12. CDC defines an unintended pregnancy as one that is either unwanted (i.e., the pregnancy occurred when no children, or no more children, were desired) or mistimed (i.e., the pregnancy occurred earlier than desired). The proportion of women at risk for unintended pregnancy who used a highly effective reversible method, known as long-acting reversible contraception (LARC), ranged from 5.5% to 18.9% for BRFSS-surveyed women and 6.9% to 30.5% for PRAMS/MIHA-surveyed women. The proportion of women not using any contraception ranged from 12.3% to 34.3% (BRFSS) and from 3.5% to 15.3% (PRAMS/MIHA). YRBS data indicated that among sexually active female high school students, use of LARC at last intercourse ranged from 1.7% to 8.4%, and use of no contraception ranged from 7.3% to 22.8%. In the context of zika preparedness, the full range of contraceptive methods approved by the Food and Drug Administration (FDA), including LARC, should be readily available and accessible for women who want to avoid or delay pregnancy. Given low rates of LARC use, states can implement strategies to remove barriers to the access and availability of LARC including high device costs, limited provider reimbursement, lack of training for providers serving women and adolescents on insertion and removal of LARC, provider lack of knowledge and misperceptions about LARC, limited availability of youth-friendly services that address adolescent confidentiality concerns, inadequate client-centered counseling, and low consumer awareness of the range of contraceptive methods available [218, 219]. To support state and territory response to the threat of zika, CDC's Interim Zika Response Plan outlined activities for vector control, clinical management of exposed pregnant women and infants, targeted communication about ZIKV transmission among women and men of reproductive age, and primary prevention of zika-related adverse pregnancy and birth outcomes by prevention of unintended pregnancies through increased access to contraception. The most highly effective, reversible contraception includes intrauterine devices and implants, known as LARC. On September 28th, 2016, the Association of Maternal and Child Health Programs (AMCHP) and CDC facilitated a meeting in Atlanta, Georgia, of representatives from 15 states to identify state-led efforts to implement seven CDC-published strategies aimed at increasing access to contraception in the context of ZIKV. Qualitative data were collected from participating jurisdictions. The number of states reporting implementation of each strategy ranged from four to 11. Participants identified numerous challenges, particularly for strategies implemented less frequently. Examples of barriers were discussed and presented with corresponding approaches to address each barrier. Addressing these barriers could facilitate increased access to contraception, which might decrease the number of unintended pregnancies affected by ZIKV [220]. Ensuring access to and promoting use of effective contraception have been identified as important strategies for preventing unintended pregnancy. The importance of ensuring resources to prevent unintended pregnancy in the context of public health emergencies was highlighted during the 2016 ZIKV outbreak when ZIKV infection during pregnancy was identified as a cause of serious birth defects. Accordingly, CDC outlined strategies for state, local, and territorial jurisdictions to consider implementing to ensure access to contraception. To update previously published contraceptive use estimates among women at risk for unintended pregnancy and to estimate the number of women with ongoing or potential need for contraceptive services, data on contraceptive use were collected during September-December 2016 through the BRFSS. Results from 21 jurisdictions indicated that most women aged 18-49 years were at risk for unintended pregnancy (range across jurisdictions = 57.4-76.8%). Estimates of the number of women with ongoing or potential need for contraceptive services ranged from 368 to 617 per 1,000 women aged 18-49 years. The percentage of women at risk for unintended pregnancy using a most or moderately effective contraceptive method ranged from 26.1% to 65.7%. Jurisdictions can use this information to estimate the number of women who might seek contraceptive services and to plan and evaluate efforts to increase contraceptive use. This information is particularly important in the context of public health emergencies, such as the recent ZIKV outbreak, which have been associated with increased risk for adverse maternal-infant outcomes and have highlighted the importance of providing women and their partners with resources to prevent unintended pregnancy [221].

ZIKV RNA has been detected in a number of body fluids, including blood, urine, saliva, and amniotic fluid, and whereas transmission associated with occupational exposure to these body fluids is theoretically possible, it has not been documented. Although there are no reports of transmission of ZIKV from infected patients to health care personnel or other patients, minimizing exposures to body fluids is important to reduce the possibility of such transmission. CDC recommends standard precautions in all health care settings to protect both health care personnel and patients from infection with ZIKV as well as from blood-borne pathogens (e.g., HIV and HCV). Because of the potential for exposure to large volumes of body fluids during the labor and delivery process and the sometimes unpredictable and fast-paced nature of obstetric care, the use of standard precautions in these settings is essential to prevent possible transmission of ZIKV from patients to health care personnel [222]. Multiple arbovirus epidemics continue to occur and challenge blood safety policy makers in non-endemic developed countries. There is new documentation of transfusion transmission of DENV and Ross River Virus (RRV), and new or increased concern about CHIKV and ZIKV. Considering that the virus causes a viremia in which 80% of infected individuals have no symptoms, the potential for transfusion transmission from an asymptomatic blood donor is high if utilizing donor screening alone without testing. Platelet units have been shown to infect two patients via transfusion in Brazil. Although there was an investigational nucleic acid test available for testing donors, not all blood centers were initially required to participate. Subsequently, the US FDA issued a guidance in August 2016 that recommended universal nucleic acid testing for the ZIKV on blood donors. Ultimately, this current global threat, as described by the WHO, will inevitably be followed by future outbreaks of other bloodborne pathogens; the principles and practices of perioperative patient blood management will reduce the risks from not only known, but also unknown risks of blood transfusion for our patients [223]. Pathogen inactivation has been shown to inactivate almost all bacterial species and several epidemic arboviruses that pose a transfusion transmission risk. The two available platelet pathogen inactivation technologies show different levels of pathogen inactivation as measured by *in vitro* infectivity assays; the clinical significance of this finding is not known. Pathogen inactivation can mitigate infectious risk and should do so more completely than other interventions such as donor questioning, donor/component recall, or donor testing. However, pathogen inactivation increases the cost of the pathogen-reduced blood component, which is a significant obstacle in the current healthcare environment. This may inhibit the ability to move forward with an effective new paradigm for blood safety that fulfills the implicit public trust in the blood system [224, 225].

There are no licensed vaccines for ZIKV; however, many vaccine platforms/approaches that have been utilized for other Flavivirus vaccines are being applied to ZIKV [226]. On the basis of previous studies, it has long been stated that 17D yellow fever vaccine generally did not induce complement-fixing (CF) antibodies, and that the presence of CF antibodies could be used in epidemiological studies to distinguish individuals infected with wild YFV from vaccinated persons. The practical significance of these studies is that they demonstrated that in a high percentage of persons with prior Flavivirus exposure, anamnestic serological responses to yellow fever vaccine result in CF antibodies similar to those induced by natural YFV infection. In Africa and tropical America, where the background of flaviviral immunity is high, it is imperative that sero-epidemiological investigations during or after yellow fever outbreaks be conducted prior to vaccination [227]. Various companies are working to develop a vaccine and antiviral medicine against ZIKV. Despite promising results, the road remains long until a vaccine or antiviral medicines are available [228]. To further complicate the matters, ZIKV is genetically similar (about 40%)

with the four serotypes of DENV, so much so that it can almost be called a fifth dengue serotype. This homology poses the risk of causing cross-reactive immune responses and subsequent antibody-dependent enhancement (ADE) of infection in case of secondary infections or for immunized individuals. All of these factors complicate the development of a single preventive vaccine candidate or a pharmacological intervention that will completely eliminate or cure ZIKV infection. A combinatorial approach including immunization and treatment might prove to be the winning strategy [229]. Until we reach a firm conclusion, past experience with another virus that causes damage to newborns offers some hope. The development and almost universal use of rubella vaccine has all but eliminated the congenital rubella syndrome in the world. Rapid development of ZIKV vaccine might well do the same for this epidemic [230-235].

Recent efforts towards the development of a vaccine have been remarkable from both the private and public sectors and include new candidate vaccines ranging from the classical live-attenuated or inactivated vaccines to more sophisticated approaches such as messenger RNA (mRNA) or genetically engineered viral platforms. Previous successes with licensed Flavivirus vaccines indicate that a protective ZIKV vaccine should be an achievable goal. Nevertheless, numerous pre- and post-licensure challenges need to be taken into account, such as the interaction of vaccine-induced immune responses with other Flaviviruses, in particular with dengue, where antibody-dependent enhancement could become an issue, and the importance of a rapid induction of protective responses during pregnancy [236]. As a result, there are currently 45 ZIKV vaccine candidates in development. Both traditional (purified inactivated, live attenuated, viral-vectored, and recombinant sub-unit) and novel (deoxy-ribonucleic acid [DNA], self-replicating RNA, and mRNA) vaccine platforms are being utilized. For emergency use, vaccines that are appropriate for women of child-bearing age (including pregnant women) are being developed. Live vaccines that may be contraindicated in pregnancy are also in development for potential inclusion in national immunization programs in childhood or pre-teenage age groups. WHO developed a target product profile for zika vaccines for use in an emergency. Although ZIKV vaccine development had a quick head start, further development may be hampered because of the inability to conduct large efficacy trials with the decline in cases globally and unpredictability of new outbreaks. Furthermore, there are complex ethical issues involved in conducting efficacy trials in pregnant women [237-239]. As evidenced from recent epidemics, both EBOV and ZIKV infections are potentially catastrophic when occurring in pregnant women. Production of efficacious vaccines has been a public health priority for both infections. Unfortunately, during the clinical trials and subsequent deployment of a vaccine for the EBOV, pregnant and lactating women were, and continue to be, excluded from receiving the life-saving vaccine. The most serious consequence of ZIKV infection, CZS, results from fetal infection during pregnancy. Thus, pregnant women have a major stake in the ongoing development of a vaccine for ZIKV. The exclusion of pregnant women from the development, clinical trials, and administration of a potential zika vaccine unfairly deprives them and their infants of the protection they need against this potentially catastrophic intrauterine infection. When creating policy about these issues, it is important to critically evaluate vaccine safety in pregnancy in the context of the substantial risk of infection for the pregnant woman and her fetus in the absence of immunization [240].

The National Institute of Allergy and Infectious Diseases (NAID), part of the National Institutes of Health (NIH), has launched a vaccine trial at the beginning of August 2016 to control ZIKV transmission: patients who received the vaccine were expected to return within 44 weeks to determine if the vaccine is safe. Results show that high levels of sexual transmission create larger cases of infection associated with the peak of infected humans arising in a shorter period of time, even when a vaccine is available in the population. However, a high level of transmission of zika from vectors to humans compared with sexual transmission represents that ZIKV will take longer to invade the population providing a window of opportunities to control its spread, for instance, through vaccination [241]. Development of new vaccines and drugs is challenging and several points particular to ZIKV infections augment this difficulty:

1) cross-reactions between ZIKV and other Flaviviruses: the impact of ZIKV vaccination on subsequent Flavivirus infections, and vice-versa, is unknown;
2) drugs against ZIKV should be safe in pregnant women; and
3) evaluation of the efficacy of vaccine and drugs against ZIKV in clinical trials phase II-IV will be complicated due to the decline of ZIKV circulation [242, 243].

A rapid response by academia, government, public health infrastructure, and industry has enabled the expedited development and testing of a suite of vaccine platforms aiming to control and eliminate ZIKV-induced disease. Analysis of key immunization and pathogenesis studies in multiple animal models, including during pregnancy, has begun to define immune correlates of protection. Nonetheless, the deployment of ZIKV vaccines, along with the confirmation of their safety and efficacy, still has major challenges, one of which is related to the waning of the epidemic [244].

TREATMENT

After the WHO declared ZIKV as a PHEIC, intense research for the development of vaccines and drugs has been undertaken, leading to the development of several candidate compounds targeting ZIKV proteins, i.e., the envelope and capsid structural proteins, the non-structural protein 3 (NS3) helicase/protease, and the NS5 methyltransferase/RNA-dependent RNA polymerase. Research for effective drugs against ZIKV is still in a very early discovery phase. Notwithstanding the intense efforts for the development of new drugs and the identification of several promising candidates by using different approaches, including computational methods, so far only a few candidates have been experimentally tested. An important caveat of anti-Flavivirus drug development is represented by the difficult of reproducing the *in vivo* microenvironment of the replication complex, which may lead to discrepancies between *in vitro* results and *in vivo* experimental evaluation. Moreover, anti-ZIKV drugs have the additional requirement of an excellent safety profile in pregnancy and ability to diffuse to different tissues, including the CNS, the testis, and the placenta [245]. Drug trials in pregnancy raise several scientific, ethical, and logistic challenges, which are compounded further in ZIKV because of limited knowledge of the disease pathophysiology and a product development pipeline in its infancy. The major challenges in choosing therapeutics to prevent congenital ZIKV disease and conducting clinical trials of these treatments must be characterized and planned for now so that clinical trials can progress expediently and effectively in the future [246]. Genomic and molecular investigations are underway to investigate ZIKV pathology and its recent enhanced pathogenicity, as well as to design safe and potent vaccines, drugs, and therapeutics. Anti-ZIKV therapeutics include drugs targeting virus entry into cells and the helicase protein, nucleosides, inhibitors of NS3 protein, small molecules, methyltransferase inhibitors, IFN, repurposed drugs, drugs designed with the aid of computers, neutralizing antibodies, convalescent serum, antibodies that limit antibody-dependent enhancement, and herbal medicines. Additionally, covalent inhibitors of viral protein expression and anti-Toll-like receptor (TLR) molecules. To counter ZIKV-associated disease, we need to make rapid progress in developing novel therapies that work effectually to inhibit ZIKV [247-249].

CONCLUSION

The worldwide invasion of arboviruses in recent decades is responsible for emerging public health threats. Some factors like climate change, urbanization, and uncontrolled population growth are fueling their widespread. Arboviruses incorporate a vast collection of genetically diverse viral pathogens including that of dengue, zika, and chikungunya. These viruses are peculiar as they are zoonotic and are a serious harm to the society, with no particular therapy to neutralize their effect. So, it is the need of the hour to develop an effective treatment against infections caused by them [250]. The CDC have developed specific molecular and serologic testing protocols and algorithms for follow-up care of suspected cases. Currently, the mainstay of management is conservative care while researchers attempt to develop a vaccine. Strategies to contain ZIKV include vector control, travel restriction for women who are pregnant or trying to become pregnant, and avoidance of mosquito bites in endemic regions of the world. The global epidemic of ZIKV infection has emerged as an important public health problem affecting pregnant women and their infants. Many questions remain regarding the risk factors, pathophysiology, epidemiology, and timing of maternal-fetal transmission and disease. These include mechanisms of fetal brain damage and microcephaly, the role of covariables, such as viral burden, duration of viremia, and host genetics, on vertical transmission, and the clinical and pathological spectrum of CZS. Additional questions include defining the potential long-term physical and neurobehavioral outcomes for infected infants, whether maternal or fetal host genetics influence the clinical outcome, and whether ZIKV infection can cause maternal morbidity. Recent advances in epidemiology, clinical medicine, pathology, and experimental studies have provided a great amount of new information regarding vertical ZIKV transmission and the mechanisms of congenital microcephaly, brain damage, and CZS in a relatively short time. However, much work still needs to be performed to more completely understand the maternal and fetal aspects of this new and emerging viral disease [251]. The future outlook regarding the current ZIKV outbreak in the Americas remains uncertain. What is certain is our need to promptly and efficiently address research gaps in our understanding of clinical outcomes from infection and environmental factors that influence emergence meanwhile improving diagnostic, therapeutic, and preventive measures against the disease [252]. There is a need to perform updated systematic reviews on ZIKV infection periodically because this epidemic is bringing up new evidence with extraordinary speed. Many challenges are still far from being solved regarding the epidemiology, case definition, clinical and laboratory diagnosis, and preventive measures. An approach using "omics" and new biomarkers for diagnosis, and a ZIKV-vaccine for treatment, might finally give us the tools to solve these challenges [253].

REFERENCES

[1] Rather, I. A., Lone, J. B., Bajpai, V. K., Paek, W. K. and Lim, J. (2017). Zika Virus: An Emerging Worldwide Threat. *Front Microbiol*, 8: 1417.

[2] Goeijenbier, M., Slobbe, L., van der Eijk, A., de Mendonça Melo, M., Koopmans, M. P. and Reusken, C. B. (2016). Zika virus and the current outbreak: an overview. *Neth J Med*, 74 (3): 104-109.

[3] Beckham, J. D., Pastula, D. M., Massey, A. and Tyler, K. L. (2016). Zika Virus as an Emerging Global Pathogen: Neurological Complications of Zika Virus. *JAMA Neurol*, 73 (7): 875-879.

[4] Benzekri, R., Belfort, R. Jr., Ventura, C. V., de Paula Freitas, B., Maia, M., Leite, M., Labetoulle, M. and Rousseau, A. (2017). Ocular manifestations of Zika virus: What we do and do not know. *J Fr Ophtalmol*, 40 (2): 138-145.

[5] Hajra, A., Bandyopadhyay, D. and Hajra, S. K. (2016). Zika Virus: A Global Threat to Humanity: A Comprehensive Review and Current Developments. *N Am J Med Sci*, 8 (3): 123-128.

[6] Yun, S. I. and Lee, Y. M. (2017). Zika virus: An emerging flavivirus. *J Microbiol*, 55 (3): 204-219.

[7] Saiz, J. C., Martín-Acebes, M. A., Bueno-Marí, R., Salomón, O. D., Villamil-Jiménez, L. C., Heukelbach, J., Alencar, C. H., Armstrong, P. K., Ortiga-Carvalho, T. M., Mendez-Otero, R., Rosado-de-Castro, P. H. and Pimentel-Coelho, P. M. (2017). Zika Virus: What Have We Learnt Since the Start of the Recent Epidemic? *Front Microbiol*, 8: 1554.

[8] D'Alò, G. L., Ciabattini, M., Zaratti, L. and Franco, E. (2016). Zika virus: a public health overview on epidemiology, clinical practice and prevention. *Ig Sanita Pubbl*, 72 (2): 161-180.

[9] Sikka, V., Chattu, V. K., Popli, R. K., Galwankar, S. C., Kelkar, D., Sawicki, S. G., Stawicki, S. P. and Papadimos, T. J. (2016). The Emergence of Zika Virus as a Global Health Security Threat: A Review and a Consensus Statement of the INDUSEM Joint working Group (JWG). *J Glob Infect Dis*, 8 (1): 3-15.

[10] Borchardt, R. A. (2016). Zika virus: A rapidly emerging infectious disease. *JAAPA*, 29 (4): 48-50.

[11] Oussayef, N. L., Pillai, S. K., Honein, M. A., Ben Beard, C., Bell, B., Boyle, C. A., Eisen, L. M., Kohl, K., Kuehnert, M. J., Lathrop, E., Martin, S. W., Martin, R., McAllister, J. C., McClune, E. P., Mead, P., Meaney-Delman, D., Petersen, B., Petersen, L. R., Polen, K. N., Powers, A. M., Redd, S. C., Sejvar, J. J., Sharp, T., Villanueva, J. and Jamieson, D. J. (2017). Zika Virus – 10 Public Health Achievements in 2016 and Future Priorities. *MMWR Morb Mortal Wkly Rep*, 65 (52): 1482-1488.

[12] Igbinosa, I. I., Rabe, I. B., Oduyebo, T. and Rasmussen, S. A. (2017). Zika Virus: Common Questions and Answers. *Am Fam Physician*, 95 (8): 507-513.

[13] Wikan, N. and Smith, D. R. (2016). Zika virus: history of a newly emerging arbovirus. *Lancet Infect Dis*, 16 (7): e119-e126.

[14] Guillier, A., Amazan, E., Aoun, A., Baubion, E. and Derancourt, C. (2017). Zika virus infection: A review. *Ann Dermatol Venereol*, 144 (8-9): 518-524.

[15] Shirley, D. T. and Nataro, J. P. (2017). Zika Virus Infection. *Pediatr Clin North Am*, 64 (4): 937-951.

[16] Kuno, G. and Chang, G. J. (2007). Full-length sequencing and genomic characterization of Bagaza, Kedougou, and Zika viruses. *Arch Virol*, 152 (4): 687-696.

[17] Pierson, T. C. and Diamond, M. S. (2018). The emergence of Zika virus and its new clinical syndromes. *Nature*, 560 (7720): 573-581.

[18] Faye, O., Freire, C. C., Iamarino, A., Faye, O., de Oliveira, J. V., Diallo, M., Zanotto, P. M. and Sall, A. A. (2014). Molecular evolution of Zika virus during its emergence in the 20th century. *PLoS Negl Trop Dis*, 8 (1): e2636.

[19] Krause, K. K., Azouz, F., Shin, O. S. and Kumar, M. (2017). Understanding the Pathogenesis of Zika Virus Infection Using Animal Models. *Immune Netw*, 17 (5): 287-297.

[20] Pawitwar, S. S., Dhar, S., Tiwari, S., Ojha, C. R., Lapierre, J., Martins, K., Rodzinski, A., Parira, T., Paudel, I., Li, J., Dutta, R. K., Silva, M. R., Kaushik, A. and El-Hage, N. (2017). Overview on the Current Status of Zika Virus Pathogenesis and Animal Related Research. *J Neuroimmune Pharmacol*, 12 (3): 371-388.

[21] Jurado, K. A., Simoni, M. K., Tang, Z., Uraki, R., Hwang, J., Householder, S., Wu, M., Lindenbach, B. D., Abrahams, V. M., Guller, S. and Fikrig, E. (2016). Zika virus productively infects primary human placenta-specific macrophages. *JCI Insight*, 1 (13): e88461.

[22] Reyes, L. and Golos, T. G. (2018). Hofbauer Cells: Their Role in Healthy and Complicated Pregnancy. *Front Immunol*, 9: 2628.

[23] Schwartz, D. A. (2017). Viral infection, proliferation, and hyperplasia of Hofbauer cells and absence of inflammation characterize the placental pathology of fetuses with congenital Zika virus infection. *Arch Gynecol Obstet*, 295 (6): 1361-1368.

[24] Sheridan, M. A., Yunusov, D., Balaraman, V., Alexenko, A. P., Yabe, S., Verjovski-Almeida, S., Schust, D. J., Franz, A. W., Sadovsky, Y., Ezashi, T. and Roberts, R. M. (2017). Vulnerability of primitive human placental trophoblast to Zika virus. *Proc Natl Acad Sci U S A*, 114 (9): E1587-E1596.

[25] El Costa, H., Gouilly, J., Mansuy, J. M., Chen, Q., Levy, C., Cartron, G., Veas, F., Al-Daccak, R., Izopet, J. and Jabrane-Ferrat, N. (2016). ZIKA virus reveals broad tissue and cell tropism during the first trimester of pregnancy. *Sci Rep*, 6: 35296.

[26] Zhang, Z. W., Li, Z. L. and Yuan, S. (2017). The Role of Secretory Autophagy in Zika Virus Transfer through the Placental Barrier. *Front Cell Infect Microbiol*, 6: 206.

[27] Delorme-Axford, E. and Klionsky, D. J. (2019). Inflammatory-dependent Sting activation induces antiviral autophagy to limit zika virus in the Drosophila brain. *Autophagy*, 15 (1): 1-3.

[28] Mawson, A. R. (2016). Pathogenesis of Zika Virus-Associated Embryopathy. *Biores Open Access*, 5 (1): 171-176.

[29] Simões E. Silva, A. C., Moreira, J. M., Romanelli, R. M. and Teixeira, A. L. (2016). Zika virus challenges for neuropsychiatry. *Neuropsychiatr Dis Treat*, 12: 1747-1760.

[30] Hickman, H. D. and Pierson, T. C. (2016). Zika in the Brain: New Models Shed Light on Viral Infection. *Trends Mol Med*, 22 (8): 639-641.

[31] Carod-Artal, F. J. (2018). Neurological complications of Zika virus infection. *Expert Rev Anti Infect Ther*, 16 (5): 399-410.

[32] Rolfe, A. J., Bosco, D. B., Wang, J., Nowakowski, R. S., Fan, J. and Ren, Y. (2016). Bioinformatic analysis reveals the expression of unique transcriptomic signatures in Zika virus infected human neural stem cells. *Cell Biosci*, 6: 42.

[33] Goodfellow, F. T., Willard, K. A., Wu, X., Scoville, S., Stice, S. L. and Brindley, M. A. (2018). Strain-Dependent Consequences of Zika Virus Infection and Differential Impact on Neural Development. *Viruses*, 10 (10): E550.

[34] Retallack, H., Di Lullo, E., Arias, C., Knopp, K. A., Laurie, M. T., Sandoval-Espinosa, C., Mancia Leon, W. R., Krencik, R., Ullian, E. M., Spatazza, J., Pollen, A. A., Mandel-Brehm, C., Nowakowski, T. J., Kriegstein, A. R. and DeRisi, J. L. (2016). Zika virus cell tropism in the developing human brain and inhibition by azithromycin. *Proc Natl Acad Sci U S A*, 113 (50): 14408-14413.

[35] Volpi, V. G., Pagani, I., Ghezzi, S., Iannacone, M., D'Antonio, M. and Vicenzi, E. (2018). Zika Virus Replication in Dorsal Root Ganglia Explants from Interferon Receptor1 Knockout Mice Causes Myelin Degeneration. *Sci Rep*, 8 (1): 10166.

[36] Saad, T., PennaeCosta, A. A., de Góes, F. V., de Freitas, M., de Almeida, J. V., de Santa Ignêz, L. J., Amancio, A. P., Alvim, R. J. and Antunes Kramberger, L. A. (2018). Neurological manifestations of congenital Zika virus infection. *Childs Nerv Syst*, (34): 73-78.

[37] Janssens, S., Schotsaert, M., Karnik, R., Balasubramaniam, V., Dejosez, M., Meissner, A., García-Sastre, A. and Zwaka, T. P.

(2018). Zika Virus Alters DNA Methylation of Neural Genes in an Organoid Model of the Developing Human Brain. *MSystems*, (3): e00219-17.

[38] Lee, J. K. and Shin, O. S. (2019). Advances in Zika Virus-Host Cell Interaction: Current Knowledge and Future Perspectives. *Int J Mol Sci*, 20 (5): E1101.

[39] Desai, S. K., Hartman, S. D., Jayarajan, S., Liu, S. and Gallicano, G. I. (2017). Zika Virus (ZIKV): a review of proposed mechanisms of transmission and associated congenital abnormalities. *Am J Stem Cells*, 6 (2): 13-22.

[40] Chakhtoura, N., Hazra, R. and Spong, C. Y. (2018). Zika virus: a public health perspective. *Curr Opin Obstet Gynecol*, 30 (2): 116-122.

[41] Faizan, M. I., Abdullah, M., Ali, S., Naqvi, I. H., Ahmed, A. and Parveen, S. (2016). Zika Virus-Induced Microcephaly and Its Possible Molecular Mechanism. *Intervirology*, 59 (3): 152-158.

[42] Zhou, K., Wang, L., Yu, D., Huang, H., Ji, H. and Mo, X. (2017). Molecular and cellular insights into Zika virus-related neuropathies. *J Neurovirol*, 23 (3): 341-346.

[43] Zorec, R., Županc, T. A. and Verkhratsky, A. (2019). Astrogliopathology in the infectious insults of the brain. *Neurosci Lett*, 689: 56-62.

[44] Geser, A., Henderson, B. E. and Christensen, S. (1970). A multipurpose serological survey in Kenya. 2. Results of arbovirus serological tests. *Bull World Health Organ*, 43 (4): 539-552.

[45] Monath, T. P., Wilson, D. C. and Casals, J. (1973). The 1970 yellow fever epidemic in Okwoga District, Benue Plateau State, Nigeria. 3. Serological responses in persons with and without pre-existing heterologous group B immunity. *Bull World Health Organ*, 49 (3): 235-244.

[46] Lanciotti, R. S., Kosoy, O. L., Laven, J. J., Velez, J. O., Lambert, A. J., Johnson, A. J., Stanfield, S. M. and Duffy, M. R. (2008). Genetic and serologic properties of Zika virus associated with an epidemic, Yap State, Micronesia, 2007. *Emerg Infect Dis*, 14 (8): 1232-1239.

[47] Hayes, E. B. (2009). Zika virus outside Africa. *Emerg Infect Dis*, 15 (9): 1347-1350.

[48] Weissenböck, H., Hubálek, Z., Bakonyi, T. and Nowotny, N. (2010). Zoonotic mosquito-borne flaviviruses: worldwide presence of agents with proven pathogenicity and potential candidates of future emerging diseases. *Vet Microbiol*, 140 (3-4): 271-280.

[49] de Laval, F., Leparc-Goffart, I., Meynard, J. B., Daubigny, H., Simon, F. and Briolant, S. (2016). Zika virus infections. *Med Sante Trop*, 26 (2): 145-150.

[50] Haddow, A. D., Schuh, A. J., Yasuda, C. Y., Kasper, M. R., Heang, V., Huy, R., Guzman, H., Tesh, R. B. and Weaver, S. C. (2012). Genetic characterization of Zika virus strains: geographic expansion of the Asian lineage. *PLoS Negl Trop Dis*, 6 (2): e1477.

[51] Ioos, S., Mallet, H. P., Leparc Goffart, I., Gauthier, V., Cardoso, T. and Herida, M. (2014). Current Zika virus epidemiology and recent epidemics. *Med Mal Infect*, 44 (7): 302-307.

[52] Choumet, V. and Desprès, P. (2015). Dengue and other flavivirus infections. *Rev Sci Tech*, 34 (2): 467-478.

[53] Fernández-Salas, I., Díaz-González, E. E., López-Gatell, H. and Alpuche-Aranda, C. (2016). Chikugunya and zika virus dissemination in the Americas: different arboviruses reflecting the same spreading routes and poor vector-control policies. *Curr Opin Infect Dis*, 29 (5): 467-475.

[54] Teixeira, M. G., Costa Mda, C., de Oliveira, W. K., Nunes, M. L. and Rodrigues, L. C. (2016). The Epidemic of Zika Virus-Related Microcephaly in Brazil: Detection, Control, Etiology, and Future Scenarios. *Am J Public Health*, 106 (4): 601-605.

[55] Paploski, I. A., Prates, A. P., Cardoso, C. W., Kikuti, M., Silva, M. M., Waller, L. A., Reis, M. G., Kitron, U. and Ribeiro, G. S. (2016). Time Lags between Exanthematous Illness Attributed to Zika Virus, Guillain-Barré Syndrome, and Microcephaly, Salvador, Brazil. *Emerg Infect Dis*, 22 (8): 1438-1444.

[56] Paixão, E. S., Barreto, F., Teixeira Mda, G., Costa Mda, C. and Rodrigues, L. C. (2016). History, Epidemiology, and Clinical

Manifestations of Zika: A Systematic Review. *Am J Public Health*, 106 (4): 606-612.

[57] Olagnier, D., Muscolini, M., Coyne, C. B., Diamond, M. S. and Hiscott, J. (2016). Mechanisms of Zika Virus Infection and Neuropathogenesis. *DNA Cell Biol*, 35 (8): 367-372.

[58] Lucchese, G. and Kanduc, D. (2016). Zika virus and autoimmunity: From microcephaly to Guillain-Barré syndrome, and beyond. *Autoimmun Rev*, 15 (8): 801-808.

[59] Journel, I., Andrécy, L. L., Metellus, D., Pierre, J. S., Faublas, R. M., Juin, S., Dismer, A. M., Fitter, D. L., Neptune, D., Laraque, M. J., Corvil, S., Pierre, M., Buteau, J., Lafontant, D., Patel, R., Lemoine, J. F., Lowrance, D. W., Charles, M., Boncy, J. and Adrien, P. (2017). Transmission of Zika Virus – Haiti, October 12, 2015-September 10, 2016. *MMWR Morb Mortal Wkly Rep*, 66 (6): 172-176.

[60] Lee, C. T., Vora, N. M., Bajwa, W., Boyd, L., Harper, S., Kass, D., Langston, A., McGibbon, E., Merlino, M., Rakeman, J. L., Raphael, M., Slavinski, S., Tran, A., Wong, R. and Varma J. K.; NYC Zika Response Team. (2016). Zika Virus Surveillance and Preparedness – New York City, 2015-2016. *MMWR Morb Mortal Wkly Rep*, 65 (24): 629-635.

[61] Healy, J. M., Burgess, M. C., Chen, T. H., Hancock, W. T., Toews, K. E., Anesi, M. S., Tulafono, R. T. Jr., Mataia, M. A., Sili, B., Solaita, J., Whelen, A. C., Sciulli, R., Gose, R. B., Uluiviti, V., Hennessey, M., Utu, F., Nua, M. T. and Fischer, M. (2016). Notes from the Field: Outbreak of Zika Virus Disease – American Samoa, 2016. *MMWR Morb Mortal Wkly Rep*, 65 (41): 1146-1147.

[62] Hennessey, M., Fischer, M. and Staples, J. E. (2016). Zika Virus Spreads to New Areas – Region of the Americas, May 2015-January 2016. *MMWR Morb Mortal Wkly Rep*, 65 (3): 55-58.

[63] Dirlikov, E., Ryff, K. R., Torres-Aponte, J., Thomas, D. L., Perez-Padilla, J., Munoz-Jordan, J., Caraballo, E. V., Garcia, M., Segarra, M. O., Malave, G., Simeone, R. M., Shapiro-Mendoza, C. K., Reyes, L. R., Alvarado-Ramy, F., Harris, A. F., Rivera, A., Major, C. G., Mayshack, M., Alvarado, L. I., Lenhart, A., Valencia-Prado, M.,

Waterman, S., Sharp, T. M. and Rivera-Garcia, B. (2016). Update: Ongoing Zika Virus Transmission – Puerto Rico, November 1, 2015-April 14, 2016. *MMWR Morb Mortal Wkly Rep*, 65 (17): 451-455.

[64] Adams, L., Bello-Pagan, M., Lozier, M., Ryff, K. R., Espinet, C., Torres, J., Perez-Padilla, J., Febo, M. F., Dirlikov, E., Martinez, A., Munoz-Jordan, J., Garcia, M., Segarra, M. O., Malave, G., Rivera, A., Shapiro-Mendoza, C., Rosinger, A., Kuehnert, M. J., Chung, K. W., Pate, L. L., Harris, A., Hemme, R. R., Lenhart, A., Aquino, G., Zaki, S., Read, J. S., Waterman, S. H., Alvarado, L. I., Alvarado-Ramy, F., Valencia-Prado, M., Thomas, D., Sharp, T. M. and Rivera-Garcia, B. (2016). Update: Ongoing Zika Virus Transmission – Puerto Rico, November 1, 2015-July 7, 2016. *MMWR Morb Mortal Wkly Rep*, 65 (30): 774-779.

[65] Lozier, M., Adams, L., Febo, M. F., Torres-Aponte, J., Bello-Pagan, M., Ryff, K. R., Munoz-Jordan, J., Garcia, M., Rivera, A., Read, J. S., Waterman, S. H., Sharp, T. M. and Rivera-Garcia, B. (2016). Incidence of Zika Virus Disease by Age and Sex – Puerto Rico, November 1, 2015-October 20, 2016. *MMWR Morb Mortal Wkly Rep*, 65 (30): 1219-1223.

[66] Thomas, D. L., Sharp, T. M., Torres, J., Armstrong, P. A., Munoz-Jordan, J., Ryff, K. R., Martinez-Quiñones, A., Arias-Berríos, J., Mayshack, M., Garayalde, G. J., Saavedra, S., Luciano, C. A., Valencia-Prado, M., Waterman, S. and Rivera-García, B. (2016). Local Transmission of Zika Virus – Puerto Rico, November 23, 2015-January 28, 2016. *MMWR Morb Mortal Wkly Rep*, 65 (6): 154-158.

[67] Armstrong, P., Hennessey, M., Adams, M., Cherry, C., Chiu, S., Harrist, A., Kwit, N., Lewis, L., McGuire, D. O., Oduyebo, T., Russell, K., Talley, P., Tanner, M. and Williams, C.; Zika Virus Response Epidemiology and Laboratory Team. (2016). Travel-Associated Zika Virus Disease Cases among U.S. Residents – United States, January 2015-February 2016. *MMWR Morb Mortal Wkly Rep*, 65 (11): 286-289.

[68] Ginier, M., Neumayr, A., Günther, S., Schmidt-Chanasit, J. and Blum, J. (2016). Zika without symptoms in returning travellers: What are the implications? *Travel Med Infect Dis*, 14 (1): 16-20.

[69] Walker, W. L., Lindsey, N. P., Lehman, J. A., Krow-Lucal, E. R., Rabe, I. B., Hills, S. L., Martin, S. W., Fischer, M. and Staples, J. E. (2016). Zika Virus Disease Cases – 50 States and the District of Columbia, January 1-July 31, 2016. *MMWR Morb Mortal Wkly Rep*, 65 (36): 983-986.

[70] Hall, V., Walker, W. L., Lindsey, N. P., Lehman, J. A., Kolsin, J., Landry, K., Rabe, I. B., Hills, S. L., Fischer, M., Staples, J. E., Gould, C. V. and Martin, S. W. (2018). Update: Noncongenital Zika Virus Disease Cases – 50 U.S. States and the District of Columbia, 2016. *MMWR Morb Mortal Wkly Rep*, 67 (9): 265-269.

[71] Ronchetti, R. and Bianco, P. M. (2016). Many doubts about the relationship between cases of microcephaly and Zika virus in Brazil. *Epidemiol Prev*, 40 (6): 466-471.

[72] Zorrilla, C. D., Mosquera, A. M., Rabionet, S. and Rivera-Viñas, J. (2016). HIV and ZIKA in Pregnancy: Parallel Stories and New Challenges. *Obstet Gynecol Int J*, 5 (6): 180.

[73] Coelho, F. C., Durovni, B., Saraceni, V., Lemos, C., Codeco, C. T., Camargo, S., de Carvalho, L. M., Bastos, L., Arduini, D., Villela, D. A. and Armstrong, M. (2016). Higher incidence of Zika in adult women than adult men in Rio de Janeiro suggests a significant contribution of sexual transmission from men to women. *Int J Infect Dis*, 51: 128-132.

[74] Nelson, B., Morrison, S., Joseph, H., Wojno, A., Lash, R. R., Haber, Y., Berro, A., Cetron, M. and Grills, A. (2016). Travel Volume to the United States from Countries and U.S. Territories with Local Zika Virus Transmission. *PLoS Curr*, 8: pii.

[75] Galindo-Fraga, A., Ochoa-Hein, E., Sifuentes-Osornio, J. and Ruiz-Palacios, G. (2015). Zika Virus: A New Epidemic on Our Doorstep. *Rev Invest Clin*, 67 (6): 329-332.

[76] Cetron, M. (2016). Revision to CDC's Zika Travel Notices: Minimal Likelihood for Mosquito-Borne Zika Virus Transmission at

Elevations Above 2,000 Meters. *MMWR Morb Mortal Wkly Rep*, 65 (10): 267-268.

[77] Lazear, H. M. and Diamond, M. S. (2016). Zika Virus: New Clinical Syndromes and Its Emergence in the Western Hemisphere. *J Virol*, 90 (10): 4864-4875.

[78] Palomo, A. M. (2016). Zika virus: An international emergency? *J Public Health Policy*, 37 (2): 133-135.

[79] Epelboin, L., Douine, M., Carles, G., Villemant, N., Nacher, M., Rousset, D., Djossou, F. and Mosnier, E. (2016). Zika virus outbreak in Latin America: what are the challenges for French Guiana in April 2016? *Bull Soc Pathol Exot*, 109 (2): 114-125.

[80] Parry, G. J., Peacey, M. and Buenz, E. J. (2016). Little risk of severe complications associated with Zika infection in New Zealand. *N Z Med J*, 129 (1440): 108-113.

[81] Doss, C. G., Siva, R., Christopher, B. P., Chakraborty, C. and Zhu, H. (2017). Zika: How safe is India? *Infect Dis Poverty*, 6 (1): 37.

[82] Ikejezie, J., Shapiro, C. N., Kim, J., Chiu, M., Almiron, M., Ugarte, C., Espinal, M. A. and Aldighieri, S. (2017). Zika Virus Transmission – Region of the Americas, May 15, 2015-December 15, 2016. *MMWR Morb Mortal Wkly Rep*, 66 (12): 329-334.

[83] Althouse, B. M., Vasilakis, N., Sall, A. A., Diallo, M., Weaver, S. C. and Hanley, K. A. (2016). Potential for Zika Virus to Establish a Sylvatic Transmission Cycle in the Americas. *PLoS Negl Trop Dis*, 10 (12): e0005055.

[84] Chowell, G., Hincapie-Palacio, D., Ospina, J., Pell, B., Tariq, A., Dahal, S., Moghadas, S., Smirnova, A., Simonsen, L. and Viboud, C. (2016). Using Phenomenological Models to Characterize Transmissibility and Forecast Patterns and Final Burden of Zika Epidemics. *PLoS Curr*, 8: pii.

[85] Ribeiro, L. S., Marques, R. E., Jesus, A. M., Almeida, R. P. and Teixeira, M. M. (2016). Zika crisis in Brazil: challenges in research and development. *Curr Opin Virol*, 18: 76-81.

[86] Shastry, S., Koenig, K. L. and, Hirshon, J. M. (2016). Zika Virus: Critical Information for Emergency Providers. *Emerg Med Clin North Am*, 34 (3): e25-e37.

[87] Liu, L. E., Dehning, M., Phipps, A., Swienton, R. E., Harris, C. A. and Klein, K. R. (2017). Clinical Update on Dengue, Chikungunya, and Zika: What We Know at the Time of Article Submission. *Disaster Med Public Health Prep*, 11 (3): 290-299.

[88] Anderson, K. B., Thomas, S. J. and Endy, T. P. (2016). The Emergence of Zika Virus: A Narrative Review. *Ann Intern Med*, 165 (3): 175-183.

[89] Jimenez, A., Shaz, B. H. and Bloch, E. M. (2017). Zika Virus and the Blood Supply: What Do We Know? *Transfus Med Rev*, 31 (1): 1-10.

[90] Avelino-Silva, V. I. and Kallas, E. G. (2018). Untold stories of the Zika virus epidemic in Brazil. *Rev Med Virol*, 28 (6): e2000.

[91] Higuera, A. and Ramírez, J. D. (2019). Molecular epidemiology of dengue, yellow fever, Zika and Chikungunya arboviruses: An update. *Acta Trop*, 190: 99-111.

[92] Marklewitz, M. and Junglen, S. (2019). Evolutionary and ecological insights into the emergence of arthropod-borne viruses. *Acta Trop*, 190: 52-58.

[93] Freeman, M. C., Coyne, C. B., Green, M., Williams, J. V. and Silva, L. A. (2019). Emerging arboviruses and implications for pediatric transplantation: A review. *Pediatr Transplant*, 23 (1): e13303.

[94] Martinez, J. D., Garza, J. A. C. and Cuellar-Barboza, A. (2019). Going Viral 2019: Zika, Chikungunya, and Dengue. *Dermatol Clin*, 37 (1): 95-105.

[95] Beigi, R. H. (2017). Emerging Infectious Diseases in Pregnancy. *Obstet Gynecol*, 129 (5): 896-906.

[96] Kakkar, F. and Boucoiran, I. (2019). The Women and Children's Infectious Diseases Center: An integrated approach to congenital infectious diseases. *Clin Invest Med*, 41 (4): E211-E212.

[97] Coyne, C. B. and Lazear, H. M. (2016). Zika virus – Reigniting the TORCH. *Nat Rev Microbiol*, 14 (11): 707-715.

[98] Frenkel, L. D., Gomez, F. and Sabahi, F. (2018). The pathogenesis of microcephaly resulting from congenital infections: why is my baby's head so small? *Eur J Clin Microbiol Infect Dis*, 37 (2): 209-226.

[99] Levine, D., Jani, J. C., Castro-Aragon, I. and Cannie, M. (2017). How Does Imaging of Congenital Zika Compare with Imaging of Other TORCH Infections? *Radiology*, 285 (3): 744-761.

[100] Martines, R. B., Bhatnagar, J., Keating, M. K., Silva-Flannery, L., Muehlenbachs, A., Gary, J., Goldsmith, C., Hale, G., Ritter, J., Rollin, D., Shieh, W. J., Luz, K. G., Ramos, A. M., Davi, H. P., Kleber de Oliveria, W., Lanciotti, R., Lambert, A. and Zaki, S. (2016). Notes from the Field: Evidence of Zika Virus Infection in Brain and Placental Tissues from Two Congenitally Infected Newborns and Two Fetal Losses – Brazil, 2015. *MMWR Morb Mortal Wkly Rep*, 65 (6): 159-160.

[101] Kleber de Oliveira, W., Cortez-Escalante, J., De Oliveira, W. T., do Carmo, G. M., Henriques, C. M., Coelho, G. E. and Araújo de França, G. V. (2016). Increase in Reported Prevalence of Microcephaly in Infants Born to Women Living in Areas with Confirmed Zika Virus Transmission During the First Trimester of Pregnancy – Brazil, 2015. *MMWR Morb Mortal Wkly Rep*, 65 (9): 242-247.

[102] Schuler-Faccini, L., Ribeiro, E. M., Feitosa, I. M., Horovitz, D. D., Cavalcanti, D. P, P.essoa, A., Doriqui, M. J., Neri, J. I., Neto, J. M., Wanderley, H. Y., Cernach, M., El-Husny, A. S., Pone, M. V., Serao, C. L. and Sanseverino, M. T.; Brazilian Medical Genetics Society – Zika Embryopathy Task Force. (2016). Possible Association between Zika Virus Infection and Microcephaly – Brazil, 2015. *MMWR Morb Mortal Wkly Rep*, 65 (3): 59-62.

[103] Ticconi, C., Pietropolli, A. and Rezza, G. (2016). Zika virus infection and pregnancy: what we do and do not know. *Pathog Glob Health*, 110 (7-8): 262-268.

[104] Miranda-Filho Dde, B., Martelli, C. M., Ximenes, R. A., Araújo, T. V., Rocha, M. A., Ramos, R. C., Dhalia, R., França, R. F., Marques

Júnior, E. T. and Rodrigues, L. C. (2016). Initial Description of the Presumed Congenital Zika Syndrome. *Am J Public Health*, 106 (4): 598-600.

[105] de Paula Freitas, B., Ventura, C. V., Maia, M. and Belfort, R. Jr. (2017). Zika virus and the eye. *Curr Opin Ophthalmol*, 28 (6): 595-599.

[106] Ventura, C. V. and Ventura, L. O. (2018). Ophthalmologic Manifestations Associated With Zika Virus Infection. *Pediatrics*, 141 (Suppl 2): S161-S166.

[107] de Oliveira Dias, J. R., Ventura, C. V., de Paula Freitas, B., Prazeres, J., Ventura, L. O., Bravo-Filho, V., Aleman, T., Ko, A. I., Zin, A., Belfort, R. Jr. and Maia, M.; Zika Virus Study Group. (2018). Zika and the Eye: Pieces of a Puzzle. *Prog Retin Eye Res*, 66: 85-106.

[108] Leal, M. C., Muniz, L. F., Ferreira, T. S., Santos, C. M., Almeida, L. C., Van Der Linden, V., Ramos, R. C., Rodrigues, L. C. and Neto, S. S. (2016). Hearing Loss in Infants with Microcephaly and Evidence of Congenital Zika Virus Infection – Brazil, November 2015-May 2016. *MMWR Morb Mortal Wkly Rep*, 65 (34): 917-919.

[109] Graham, K. A., Fox, D. J., Talati, A., Pantea, C., Brady, L., Carter, S. L., Friedenberg, E., Vora, N. M., Browne, M. L. and Lee, C. T. (2017). Prevalence and Clinical Attributes of Congenital Microcephaly – New York, 2013-2015. *MMWR Morb Mortal Wkly Rep*, 66 (5): 125-129.

[110] Satterfield-Nash, A., Kotzky, K., Allen, J., Bertolli, J., Moore, C. A., Pereira, I. O., Pessoa, A., Melo, F., Santelli, A. C. F. E. S., Boyle, C. A. and Peacock, G. (2017). Health and Development at Age 19-24 Months of 19 Children Who Were Born with Microcephaly and Laboratory Evidence of Congenital Zika Virus Infection During the 2015 Zika Virus Outbreak – Brazil, 2017. *MMWR Morb Mortal Wkly Rep*, 66 (49): 1347-1351.

[111] van der Linden, V., Pessoa, A., Dobyns, W., Barkovich, A. J., Júnior, H. V., Filho, E. L., Ribeiro, E. M., Leal, M. C., Coimbra, P. P., Aragão, M. F., Verçosa, I., Ventura, C., Ramos, R. C., Cruz, D. D., Cordeiro, M. T., Mota, V. M., Dott, M., Hillard, C. and Moore,

C. A. (2016). Description of 13 Infants Born During October 2015-January 2016 With Congenital Zika Virus Infection Without Microcephaly at Birth – Brazil. *MMWR Morb Mortal Wkly Rep*, 65 (47): 1343-1348.

[112] Krauer, F., Riesen, M., Reveiz, L., Oladapo, O. T., Martínez-Vega, R., Porgo, T. V., Haefliger, A., Broutet, N. J. and Low, N.; WHO Zika Causality Working Group. (2017). Zika Virus Infection as a Cause of Congenital Brain Abnormalities and Guillain-Barré Syndrome: Systematic Review. *PLoS Med*, 14 (1): e1002203.

[113] Simeone, R. M., Shapiro-Mendoza, C. K., Meaney-Delman, D., Petersen, E. E., Galang, R. R., Oduyebo, T., Rivera-Garcia, B., Valencia-Prado, M., Newsome, K. B., Pérez-Padilla, J., Williams, T. R., Biggerstaff, M., Jamieson, D. J. and Honein, M. A.; Zika and Pregnancy Working Group. (2016). Possible Zika Virus Infection among Pregnant Women – United States and Territories, May 2016. *MMWR Morb Mortal Wkly Rep*, 65 (20): 514-519.

[114] Cragan, J. D., Mai, C. T., Petersen, E. E., Liberman, R. F., Forestieri, N. E., Stevens, A. C., Delaney, A., Dawson, A. L., Ellington, S. R., Shapiro-Mendoza, C. K., Dunn, J. E., Higgins, C. A., Meyer, R. E., Williams, T., Polen, K. N., Newsome, K., Reynolds, M., Isenburg, J., Gilboa, S. M., Meaney-Delman, D. M., Moore, C. A., Boyle, C. A. and Honein, M. A. (2017). Baseline Prevalence of Birth Defects Associated with Congenital Zika Virus Infection – Massachusetts, North Carolina, and Atlanta, Georgia, 2013-2014. *MMWR Morb Mortal Wkly Rep*, 66 (8): 219-222.

[115] Tutiven, J. L., Pruden, B. T., Banks, J. S., Stevenson, M. and Birnbach, D. J. (2017). Zika Virus: Obstetric and Pediatric Anesthesia Considerations. *Anesth Analg*, 124 (6): 1918-1929.

[116] Cuevas, E. L., Tong, V. T., Rozo, N., Valencia, D., Pacheco, O., Gilboa, S. M., Mercado, M., Renquist, C. M., González, M., Ailes, E. C., Duarte, C., Godoshian, V., Sancken, C. L., Turca, A. M., Calles, D. L., Ayala, M., Morgan, P., Perez, E. N., Bonilla, H. Q., Gomez, R. C., Estupiñan, A. C., Gunturiz, M. L., Meaney-Delman, D., Jamieson, D. J., Honein, M. A. and Martínez, M. L. (2016).

Preliminary Report of Microcephaly Potentially Associated with Zika Virus Infection During Pregnancy – Colombia, January-November 2016. *MMWR Morb Mortal Wkly Rep*, 65 (49): 1409-1413.

[117] Hall, N. B., Broussard, K., Evert, N. and Canfield, M. (2017). Notes from the Field: Zika Virus-Associated Neonatal Birth Defects Surveillance – Texas, January 2016-July 2017. *MMWR Morb Mortal Wkly Rep*, 66 (31): 835-836.

[118] Reynolds, M. R., Jones, A. M., Petersen, E. E., Lee, E. H., Rice, M. E., Bingham, A., Ellington, S. R., Evert, N., Reagan-Steiner, S., Oduyebo, T., Brown, C. M., Martin, S., Ahmad, N., Bhatnagar, J., Macdonald, J., Gould, C., Fine, A. D., Polen, K. D., Lake-Burger, H., Hillard, C. L., Hall, N., Yazdy, M. M., Slaughter, K., Sommer, J. N., Adamski, A., Raycraft, M., Fleck-Derderian, S., Gupta, J., Newsome, K., Baez-Santiago, M., Slavinski, S., White, J. L., Moore, C. A., Shapiro-Mendoza, C. K., Petersen, L., Boyle, C., Jamieson, D. J., Meaney-Delman, D. and Honein, M. A.; U.S. Zika Pregnancy Registry Collaboration. (2017). Vital Signs: Update on Zika Virus-Associated Birth Defects and Evaluation of All U.S. Infants with Congenital Zika Virus Exposure – U.S. Zika Pregnancy Registry, 2016. *MMWR Morb Mortal Wkly Rep*, 66 (13): 366-373.

[119] Delaney, A., Mai, C., Smoots, A., Cragan, J., Ellington, S., Langlois, P., Breidenbach, R., Fornoff, J., Dunn, J., Yazdy, M., Scotto-Rosato, N., Sweatlock, J., Fox, D., Palacios, J., Forestieri, N., Leedom, V., Smiley, M., Nance, A., Lake-Burger, H., Romitti, P., Fall, C., Prado, M. V., Barton, J., Bryan, J. M., Arias, W., Brown, S. V., Kimura, J., Mann, S., Martin, B., Orantes, L., Taylor, A., Nahabedian, J., Akosa, A., Song, Z., Martin, S., Ramlal, R., Shapiro-Mendoza, C., Isenburg, J., Moore, C. A., Gilboa, S. and Honein, M. A. (2018). Population-Based Surveillance of Birth Defects Potentially Related to Zika Virus Infection – 15 States and U.S. Territories, 2016. *MMWR Morb Mortal Wkly Rep*, 67 (3): 91-96.

[120] Rice, M. E., Galang, R. R., Roth, N. M., Ellington, S. R., Moore, C. A., Valencia-Prado, M., Ellis, E. M., Tufa, A. J., Taulung, L. A.,

Alfred, J. M., Pérez-Padilla, J., Delgado-López, C. A., Zaki, S. R., Reagan-Steiner, S., Bhatnagar, J., Nahabedian, J. F. 3rd, Reynolds, M. R., Yeargin-Allsopp, M., Viens, L. J., Olson, S. M., Jones, A. M., Baez-Santiago, M. A., Oppong-Twene, P., VanMaldeghem, K., Simon, E. L., Moore, J. T., Polen, K. D., Hillman, B., Ropeti, R., Nieves-Ferrer, L., Marcano-Huertas, M., Masao, C. A., Anzures, E. J., Hansen, R. L. Jr., Pérez-Gonzalez, S. I., Espinet-Crespo, C. P., Luciano-Román, M., Shapiro-Mendoza, C. K., Gilboa, S. M. and Honein, M. A. (2018). Vital Signs: Zika-Associated Birth Defects and Neurodevelopmental Abnormalities Possibly Associated with Congenital Zika Virus Infection – U.S. Territories and Freely Associated States, 2018. *MMWR Morb Mortal Wkly Rep*, 67 (31): 858-867.

[121] Shapiro-Mendoza, C. K., Rice, M. E., Galang, R. R., Fulton, A. C., VanMaldeghem, K., Prado, M. V., Ellis, E., Anesi, M. S., Simeone, R. M., Petersen, E. E., Ellington, S. R., Jones, A. M., Williams, T., Reagan-Steiner, S., Perez-Padilla, J., Deseda, C. C., Beron, A., Tufa, A. J., Rosinger, A., Roth, N. M., Green, C., Martin, S., Lopez, C. D., deWilde, L., Goodwin, M., Pagano, H. P., Mai, C. T., Gould, C., Zaki, S., Ferrer, L. N., Davis, M. S., Lathrop, E., Polen, K., Cragan, J. D., Reynolds, M., Newsome, K. B., Huertas, M. M., Bhatangar, J., Quiñones, A. M., Nahabedian, J. F., Adams, L., Sharp, T. M., Hancock, W. T., Rasmussen, S. A., Moore, C. A., Jamieson, D. J., Munoz-Jordan, J. L., Garstang, H., Kambui, A., Masao, C., Honein, M. A. and Meaney-Delman, D.; Zika Pregnancy and Infant Registries Working Group. (2017). Pregnancy Outcomes after Maternal Zika Virus Infection During Pregnancy – U.S. Territories, January 1, 2016-April 25, 2017. *MMWR Morb Mortal Wkly Rep*, 66 (23): 615-621.

[122] Petersen, E. E., Staples, J. E., Meaney-Delman, D., Fischer, M., Ellington, S. R., Callaghan, W. M. and Jamieson, D. J. (2016). Interim Guidelines for Pregnant Women during a Zika Virus Outbreak – United States, 2016. *MMWR Morb Mortal Wkly Rep*, 65 (2): 30-33.

[123] Oduyebo, T., Petersen, E. E., Rasmussen, S. A., Mead, P. S., Meaney-Delman, D., Renquist, C. M., Ellington, S. R., Fischer, M., Staples, J. E., Powers, A. M., Villanueva, J., Galang, R. R., Dieke, A., Muñoz, J. L., Honein, M. A. and Jamieson, D. J. (2016). Update: Interim Guidelines for Health Care Providers Caring for Pregnant Women and Women of Reproductive Age with Possible Zika Virus Exposure – United States, 2016. *MMWR Morb Mortal Wkly Rep*, 65 (5): 122-127.

[124] Petersen, E. E., Polen, K. N., Meaney-Delman, D., Ellington, S. R., Oduyebo, T., Cohn, A., Oster, A. M., Russell, K., Kawwass, J. F., Karwowski, M. P., Powers, A. M., Bertolli, J., Brooks, J. T., Kissin, D., Villanueva, J., Muñoz-Jordan, J., Kuehnert, M., Olson, C. K., Honein, M. A., Rivera, M., Jamieson, D. J. and Rasmussen, S. A. (2016). Update: Interim Guidance for Health Care Providers Caring for Women of Reproductive Age with Possible Zika Virus Exposure – United States, 2016. *MMWR Morb Mortal Wkly Rep*, 65 (12): 315-322.

[125] Oduyebo, T., Igbinosa, I., Petersen, E. E., Polen, K. N., Pillai, S. K., Ailes, E. C., Villanueva, J. M., Newsome, K., Fischer, M., Gupta, P. M., Powers, A. M., Lampe, M., Hills, S., Arnold, K. E., Rose, L. E., Shapiro-Mendoza, C. K., Beard, C. B., Muñoz, J. L., Rao, C. Y., Meaney-Delman, D., Jamieson, D. J. and Honein, M. A. (2016). Update: Interim Guidance for Health Care Providers Caring for Pregnant Women with Possible Zika Virus Exposure – United States, July 2016. *MMWR Morb Mortal Wkly Rep*, 65 (29): 739-744.

[126] Oduyebo, T., Polen, K. D., Walke, H. T., Reagan-Steiner, S., Lathrop, E., Rabe, I. B., Kuhnert-Tallman, W. L., Martin, S. W., Walker, A. T., Gregory, C. J., Ades, E. W., Carroll, D. S., Rivera, M., Perez-Padilla, J., Gould, C., Nemhauser, J. B., Ben Beard, C., Harcourt, J. L., Viens, L., Johansson, M., Ellington, S. R., Petersen, E., Smith, L. A., Reichard, J., Munoz-Jordan, J., Beach, M. J., Rose, D. A., Barzilay, E., Noonan-Smith, M., Jamieson, D. J., Zaki, S. R., Petersen, L. R., Honein, M. A. and Meaney-Delman, D. (2017). Update: Interim Guidance for Health Care Providers Caring for

Pregnant Women with Possible Zika Virus Exposure – United States (Including U.S. Territories), July 2017. *MMWR Morb Mortal Wkly Rep*, 66 (29): 781-793.

[127] Millichap, J. G. (2016). Zika Virus Infection and Microcephaly. *Pediatr Neurol Briefs*, 30 (1): 8.

[128] Meaney-Delman, D., Hills, S. L., Williams, C., Galang, R. R., Iyengar, P., Hennenfent, A. K., Rabe, I. B., Panella, A., Oduyebo, T., Honein, M. A., Zaki, S., Lindsey, N., Lehman, J. A., Kwit, N., Bertolli, J., Ellington, S., Igbinosa, I., Minta, A. A., Petersen, E. E., Mead, P., Rasmussen, S. A. and Jamieson, D. J. (2016). Zika Virus Infection among U.S. Pregnant Travelers – August 2015-February 2016. *MMWR Morb Mortal Wkly Rep*, 65 (8): 211-214.

[129] Fleming-Dutra, K. E., Nelson, J. M., Fischer, M., Staples, J. E., Karwowski, M. P., Mead, P., Villanueva, J., Renquist, C. M., Minta, A. A., Jamieson, D. J., Honein, M. A., Moore, C. A. and Rasmussen, S. A. (2016). Update: Interim Guidelines for Health Care Providers Caring for Infants and Children with Possible Zika Virus Infection – United States, February 2016. *MMWR Morb Mortal Wkly Rep*, 65 (7): 182-187.

[130] Russell, K., Oliver, S. E., Lewis, L., Barfield, W. D., Cragan, J., Meaney-Delman, D., Staples, J. E., Fischer, M., Peacock, G., Oduyebo, T., Petersen, E. E., Zaki, S., Moore, C. A. and Rasmussen, S. A.; Contributors. (2016). Update: Interim Guidance for the Evaluation and Management of Infants with Possible Congenital Zika Virus Infection – United States, August 2016. *MMWR Morb Mortal Wkly Rep*, 65 (33): 870-878.

[131] Goodman, A. B., Dziuban, E. J., Powell, K., Bitsko, R. H., Langley, G., Lindsey, N., Franks, J. L., Russell, K., Dasgupta, S., Barfield, W. D., Odom, E., Kahn, E., Martin, S., Fischer, M. and Staples, J. E. (2016). Characteristics of Children Aged <18 Years with Zika Virus Disease Acquired Postnatally – U.S. States, January 2015-July 2016. *MMWR Morb Mortal Wkly Rep*, 65 (39): 1082-1085.

[132] Adachi, K. and Nielsen-Saines, K. (2018). Zika clinical updates: implications for pediatrics. *Curr Opin Pediatr*, 30 (1): 105-116.

[133] Metcalf, C. J. and Barrett, A. (2016). Invasion Dynamics of Teratogenic Infections in Light of Rubella Control: Implications for Zika Virus. *PLoS Curr*, 8: pii.

[134] Burd, I. and Griffin, D. (2016). The chasm between public health and reproductive research: what history tells us about Zika virus. *J Assist Reprod Genet*, 33 (4): 439-440.

[135] Cordeiro, C. N., Bano, R., Washington Cross, C. I. and Segars, J. H. (2017). Zika virus and assisted reproduction. *Curr Opin Obstet Gynecol*, 29 (3): 175-179.

[136] Dubaut, J. P., Agudelo Higuita, N. I. and Quaas, A. M. (2017). Impact of Zika virus for infertility specialists: current literature, guidelines, and resources. *J Assist Reprod Genet*, 34 (10): 1237-1250.

[137] Kwak-Kim, J., Song, J., Kim, M. W. and Gilman-Sachs, A. (2017). Zika virus infection and biological treatment for reproductive medicine. *Am J Reprod Immunol*, 77 (2).

[138] Gharbaran, R. and Somenarain, L. (2019). Putative Cellular and Molecular Roles of Zika Virus in Fetal and Pediatric Neuropathologies. *Pediatr Dev Pathol*, 22 (1): 5-21.

[139] Duarte, E. C., Garcia, L. P., de Araújo, W. N. and Velez, M. P. (2017). Outcomes of Zika virus infection during pregnancy: contributions to the debate on the efficiency of cohort studies. *BMC Public Health*, 17 (1): 924.

[140] Eggo, R. M. and Kucharski, A. J. (2018). Expected Duration of Adverse Pregnancy Outcomes after Zika Epidemic. *Emerg Infect Dis*, 24 (1).

[141] Mohr, E. L. (2018). Modeling Zika Virus-Associated Birth Defects in Nonhuman Primates. *J Pediatric Infect Dis Soc*, 7 (suppl_2): S60-S66.

[142] Chibueze, E. C., Tirado, V., Lopes, K. D., Balogun, O. O., Takemoto, Y., Swa, T., Dagvadorj, A., Nagata, C., Morisaki, N., Menendez, C., Ota, E., Mori, R. and Oladapo, O. T. (2017). Zika virus infection in pregnancy: a systematic review of disease course and complications. *Reprod Health*, 14 (1): 28.

[143] Meaney-Delman, D., Rasmussen, S. A., Staples, J. E., Oduyebo, T., Ellington, S. R., Petersen, E. E., Fischer, M. and Jamieson, D. J. (2016). Zika Virus and Pregnancy: What Obstetric Health Care Providers Need to Know. *Obstet Gynecol*, 127 (4): 642-648.

[144] Zanluca, C., de Noronha, L. and Duarte Dos Santos, C. N. (2018). Maternal-fetal transmission of the zika virus: An intriguing interplay. *Tissue Barriers*, 6 (1): e1402143.

[145] Walker, C. L., Little, M. E., Roby, J. A., Armistead, B., Gale, M. Jr., Rajagopal, L., Nelson, B. R., Ehinger, N., Mason, B., Nayeri, U., Curry, C. L. and Adams Waldorf, K. M. (2019). Zika virus and the nonmicrocephalic fetus: why we should still worry. *Am J Obstet Gynecol*, 220 (1): 45-56.

[146] Sutarjono, B. (2019). Can We Better Understand How Zika Leads to Microcephaly? A Systematic Review of the Effects of the Zika Virus on Human Brain Organoids. *J Infect Dis*, 219 (5): 734-745.

[147] Majolo, F., Marinowic, D. R., Moura, A. Á., Machado, D. C. and da Costa, J. C. (2019). Use of induced pluripotent stem cells (iPSCs) and cerebral organoids in modeling the congenital infection and neuropathogenesis induced by Zika virus. *J Med Virol*, 91 (4): 525-532.

[148] Fernandes, K. M., Tomé, H. V. V., Miranda, F. R., Gonçalves, W. G., Pascini, T. V., Serrão, J. E. and Martins, G. F. (2019). Aedes aegypti larvae treated with spinosad produce adults with damaged midgut and reduced fecundity. *Chemosphere*, 221: 464-470.

[149] Pyzocha, N. J., Chinchen, S. E. and Maurer, D. M. (2017). Zany Over Zika Virus: An Overview of Diagnosis and Treatment Modalities. *Curr Sports Med Rep*, 16 (2): 109-113.

[150] Rabe, I. B., Staples, J. E., Villanueva, J., Hummel, K. B., Johnson, J. A., Rose, L., Hills, S., Wasley, A., Fischer, M. and Powers, A. M. (2016). Interim Guidance for Interpretation of Zika Virus Antibody Test Results. *MMWR Morb Mortal Wkly Rep*, 65 (21): 543-546.

[151] Bell, S. G. (2017). Laboratory Evaluation of Infants with Possible Congenital Zika Virus Infection. *Neonatal Netw*, 36 (2): 103-106.

[152] Eppes, C., Rac, M., Dunn, J., Versalovic, J., Murray, K. O., Suter, M. A., Sanz Cortes, M., Espinoza, J., Seferovic, M. D., Lee, W., Hotez, P., Mastrobattista, J., Clark, S. L., Belfort, M. A. and Aagaard, K. M. (2017). Testing for Zika virus infection in pregnancy: key concepts to deal with an emerging epidemic. *Am J Obstet Gynecol*, 216 (3): 209-225.

[153] Theel, E. S. and Hata, D. J. (2018). Diagnostic Testing for Zika Virus: a Postoutbreak Update. *J Clin Microbiol*, 56 (4): e01972-17.

[154] Lin, K. W., Kraemer, J. D., Piltch-Loeb, R. and Stoto, M. A. (2018). The Complex Interpretation and Management of Zika Virus Test Results. *J Am Board Fam Med*, 31 (6): 924-930.

[155] Peters, R. and Stevenson, M. (2019). Zika virus diagnosis: challenges and solutions. *Clin Microbiol Infect*, 25 (2): 142-146.

[156] Carod-Artal, F. J. (2016). Epidemiology and neurological complications of infection by the Zika virus: a new emerging neurotropic virus. *Rev Neurol*, 62 (7): 317-328.

[157] Bonaldo, M. C., Ribeiro, I. P., Lima, N. S., Dos Santos, A. A., Menezes, L. S., da Cruz, S. O., de Mello, I. S., Furtado, N. D., de Moura, E. E., Damasceno, L., da Silva, K. A., de Castro, M. G., Gerber, A. L., de Almeida, L. G., Lourenço-de-Oliveira, R., Vasconcelos, A. T. and Brasil, P. (2016). Isolation of Infective Zika Virus from Urine and Saliva of Patients in Brazil. *PLoS Negl Trop Dis*, 10 (6): e0004816.

[158] Dudley, D. M., Aliota, M. T., Mohr, E. L., Weiler, A. M., Lehrer-Brey, G., Weisgrau, K. L., Mohns, M. S., Breitbach, M. E., Rasheed, M. N., Newman, C. M., Gellerup, D. D., Moncla, L. H., Post, J., Schultz-Darken, N., Schotzko, M. L., Hayes, J. M., Eudailey, J. A., Moody, M. A., Permar, S. R., O'Connor, S. L., Rakasz, E. G., Simmons, H. A., Capuano, S., Golos, T. G., Osorio, J. E., Friedrich, T. C. and O'Connor, D. H. (2016). A rhesus macaque model of Asian-lineage Zika virus infection. *Nat Commun*, 7:12204.

[159] Rossi, S. L. and Vasilakis, N. (2016). Modeling Zika Virus Infection in Mice. *Cell Stem Cell*, 19 (1): 4-6.

[160] Shah, A. and Kumar, A. (2016). Zika Virus Infection and Development of a Murine Model. *Neurotox Res*, 30 (2): 131-134.

[161] Staples, J. E., Dziuban, E. J., Fischer, M., Cragan, J. D., Rasmussen, S. A., Cannon, M. J., Frey, M. T., Renquist, C. M., Lanciotti, R. S., Muñoz, J. L., Powers, A. M., Honein, M. A. and Moore, C. A. (2016). Interim Guidelines for the Evaluation and Testing of Infants with Possible Congenital Zika Virus Infection – United States, 2016. *MMWR Morb Mortal Wkly Rep*, 65 (3): 63-67.

[162] Adebanjo, T., Godfred-Cato, S., Viens, L., Fischer, M., Staples, J. E., Kuhnert-Tallman, W., Walke, H., Oduyebo, T., Polen, K., Peacock, G., Meaney-Delman, D., Honein, M. A., Rasmussen, S. A. and Moore, C. A.; Contributors. (2017). Update: Interim Guidance for the Diagnosis, Evaluation, and Management of Infants with Possible Congenital Zika Virus Infection – United States, October 2017. *MMWR Morb Mortal Wkly Rep*, 66 (41): 1089-1099.

[163] Dasgupta, S., Reagan-Steiner, S., Goodenough, D., Russell, K., Tanner, M., Lewis, L., Petersen, E. E., Powers, A. M., Kniss, K., Meaney-Delman, D., Oduyebo, T., O'Leary, D., Chiu, S., Talley, P., Hennessey, M., Hills, S., Cohn, A. and Gregory, C.; Zika Virus Response Epidemiology and Laboratory Team. (2016). Patterns in Zika Virus Testing and Infection, by Report of Symptoms and Pregnancy Status – United States, January 3-March 5, 2016. *MMWR Morb Mortal Wkly Rep*, 65 (15): 395-399.

[164] Madad, S. S., Masci, J., Cagliuso, N. V. Sr. and Allen, M. (2016). Preparedness for Zika Virus Disease – New York City, 2016. *MMWR Morb Mortal Wkly Rep*, 65 (42): 1161-1165.

[165] Hancock, W. T., Soeters, H. M., Hills, S. L., Link-Gelles, R., Evans, M. E., Daley, W. R., Piercefield, E., Anesi, M. S., Mataia, M. A., Uso, A. M., Sili, B., Tufa, A. J., Solaita, J., Irvin-Barnwell, E., Meaney-Delman, D., Wilken, J., Weidle, P., Toews, K. E., Walker, W., Talboy, P. M., Gallo, W. K., Krishna, N., Laws, R. L., Reynolds, M. R., Koneru, A. and Gould, C. V. (2017). Establishing a Timeline to Discontinue Routine Testing of Asymptomatic Pregnant Women

for Zika Virus Infection – American Samoa, 2016-2017. *MMWR Morb Mortal Wkly Rep*, 66 (11): 299-301.

[166] Braga, J. U., Bressan, C., Dalvi, A. P. R., Calvet, G. A., Daumas, R. P., Rodrigues, N., Wakimoto, M., Nogueira, R. M. R., Nielsen-Saines, K., Brito, C., Bispo de Filippis, A. M. and Brasil, P. (2017). Accuracy of Zika virus disease case definition during simultaneous Dengue and Chikungunya epidemics. *PLoS One*, 12 (6): e0179725.

[167] Koenig, K. L., Almadhyan, A. and Burns, M. J. (2016). Identify-Isolate-Inform: A Tool for Initial Detection and Management of Zika Virus Patients in the Emergency Department. *West J Emerg Med*, 17 (3): 238-244.

[168] Keighley, C. L., Saunderson, R. B., Kok, J. and Dwyer, D. E. (2015). Viral exanthems. *Curr Opin Infect Dis*, 28 (2): 139-150.

[169] Ritter, J. M., Martines, R. B. and Zaki, S. R. (2017). Zika Virus: Pathology from the Pandemic. *Arch Pathol Lab Med*, 141 (1): 49-59.

[170] Reagan-Steiner, S., Simeone, R., Simon, E., Bhatnagar, J., Oduyebo, T., Free, R., Denison, A. M., Rabeneck, D. B., Ellington, S., Petersen, E., Gary, J., Hale, G., Keating, M. K., Martines, R. B., Muehlenbachs, A., Ritter, J., Lee, E., Davidson, A., Conners, E., Scotland, S., Sandhu, K., Bingham, A., Kassens, E., Smith, L., St George, K., Ahmad, N., Tanner, M., Beavers, S., Miers, B., VanMaldeghem, K., Khan, S., Rabe, I., Gould, C., Meaney-Delman, D., Honein, M. A., Shieh, W. J., Jamieson, D. J., Fischer, M. and Zaki, S. R.; U.S. Zika Pregnancy Registry Collaboration; Zika Virus Response Epidemiology and Surveillance Task Force Pathology Team. (2017). Evaluation of Placental and Fetal Tissue Specimens for Zika Virus Infection – 50 States and District of Columbia, January-December, 2016. *MMWR Morb Mortal Wkly Rep*, 66 (24): 636-643.

[171] Moore, C. A., Staples, J. E., Dobyns, W. B., Pessoa, A., Ventura, C. V., Fonseca, E. B., Ribeiro, E. M., Ventura, L. O., Neto, N. N., Arena, J. F. and Rasmussen, S. A. (2017). Characterizing the Pattern of Anomalies in Congenital Zika Syndrome for Pediatric Clinicians. *JAMA Pediatr*, 171 (3): 288-295.

[172] Chimelli, L. and Avvad-Portari, E. (2018). Congenital Zika virus infection: a neuropathological review. *Childs Nerv Syst*, 34 (1): 95-99.

[173] Robinson, J. L. (2017). Zika virus: What does a physician caring for children in Canada need to know? *Paediatr Child Health*, 22 (1): 48-55.

[174] Chervenak, F. A., Jeanty, P., Cantraine, F., Chitkara, U., Venus, I., Berkowitz, R. L. and Hobbins, J. C. (1984). The diagnosis of fetal microcephaly. *Am J Obstet Gynecol*, 149 (5): 512-517.

[175] Gelber, S. E., Grünebaum, A. and Chervenak, F. A. (2017). Prenatal screening for microcephaly: an update after three decades. *J Perinat Med*, 45 (2): 167-170.

[176] Mace, P., Milh, M., Girard, N., Sigaudy, S. and Quarello, E. (2017). How to deal with a fetal head circumference lower than the third percentile? *Gynecol Obstet Fertil Senol*, 45 (9): 491-511.

[177] de Souza, A. S., de Oliveira-Szjenfeld, P. S., de Oliveira Melo, A. S., de Souza, L. A. M., Batista, A. G. M. and Tovar-Moll, F. (2018). Imaging findings in congenital Zika virus infection syndrome: an update. *Childs Nerv Syst*, 34 (1): 85-93.

[178] Cavalheiro, S., Lopez, A., Serra, S., Da Cunha, A., da Costa, M. D., Moron, A. and Lederman, H. M. (2016). Microcephaly and Zika virus: neonatal neuroradiological aspects. *Childs Nerv Syst*, 32 (6): 1057-1060.

[179] Araujo Júnior, E., Carvalho, F. H., Tonni, G. and Werner, H. (2017). Prenatal imaging findings in fetal Zika virus infection. *Curr Opin Obstet Gynecol*, 29 (2): 95-105.

[180] Vouga, M. and Baud, D. (2016). Imaging of congenital Zika virus infection: the route to identification of prognostic factors. *Prenat Diagn*, 36 (9): 799-811.

[181] Alvarado-Socarras, J. L., Idrovo, Á. J., Contreras-García, G. A., Rodriguez-Morales, A. J., Audcent, T. A., Mogollon-Mendoza, A. C. and Paniz-Mondolfi, A. (2018). Congenital microcephaly: A diagnostic challenge during Zika epidemics. *Travel Med Infect Dis*, 23: 14-20.

[182] Depoux, A., Philibert, A., Rabier, S., Philippe, H. J., Fontanet, A. and Flahault, A. (2018). A multi-faceted pandemic: a review of the state of knowledge on the Zika virus. *Public Health Rev*, 39: 10.

[183] Villa, R. (2016). Zika, or the burden of uncertainty. *Clin Ter*, 167 (1): 7-9.

[184] Harris, L. H., Silverman, N. S. and Marshall, M. F. (2016). The Paradigm of the Paradox: Women, Pregnant Women, and the Unequal Burdens of the Zika Virus Pandemic. *Am J Bioeth*, 16 (5): 1-4.

[185] Rasanathan, J. J., MacCarthy, S., Diniz, D., Torreele, E. and Gruskin, S. (2017). Engaging Human Rights in the Response to the Evolving Zika Virus Epidemic. *Am J Public Health*, 107 (4): 525-531.

[186] Alfaro-Murillo, J. A., Parpia, A. S., Fitzpatrick, M. C., Tamagnan, J. A., Medlock, J., Ndeffo-Mbah, M. L., Fish, D., Ávila-Agüero, M. L., Marín, R., Ko, A. I. and Galvani, A. P. (2016). A Cost-Effectiveness Tool for Informing Policies on Zika Virus Control. *PLoS Negl Trop Dis*, 10 (5): e0004743.

[187] Tambo, E., Madjou, G., Khayeka-Wandabwa, C., Olalubi, O. A., Chengho, C. F. and Khater, E. I. M. (2017). Ethical, legal and societal considerations on Zika virus epidemics complications in scaling-up prevention and control strategies. *Philos Ethics Humanit Med*, 12 (1): 3.

[188] Gyawali, N., Bradbury, R. S. and Taylor-Robinson, A. W. (2016). The global spread of Zika virus: is public and media concern justified in regions currently unaffected? *Infect Dis Poverty*, 5: 37.

[189] Johnson, S. R. (2016). Zika outbreak puts focus back on fight over abortion access. *Mod Healthc*, 46 (34): 12.

[190] de Campos, T. C. (2017). Zika, public health, and the distraction of abortion. *Med Health Care Philos*, 20 (3): 443-446.

[191] Valente, P. K. (2018). Zika and Reproductive Rights in Brazil: Challenge to the Right to Health. *Am J Public Health*, 107 (9): 1376-1380.

[192] Esquilín-Rivera, I. O., Reyes-Báez, G. and Pérez-Torres, R. (2018). Ethical Issues during Zika Epidemic in Puerto Rico and the Americas. *P R Health Sci J*, 37 (Special Issue): S41-S44.

[193] Rabionet, S. E., Zorrilla, C. D., Rivera-Viñas, J. I. and Guerra-Sanchez, Y. (2018). Pregnancy and Zika: The Quest for Quality Care and Reproductive Justice. *P R Health Sci J*, 37 (Special Issue): S45-S50.

[194] Vélez, A. C. and Diniz, S. G. (2016). Inequality, Zika epidemics, and the lack of reproductive rights in Latin America. *Reprod Health Matters*, 24 (48): 57-61.

[195] Diniz, D., Gumieri, S., Bevilacqua, B. G., Cook, R. J. and Dickens, B. M. (2017). Zika virus infection in Brazil and human rights obligations. *Int J Gynaecol Obstet*, 136 (1): 105-110.

[196] Towers, V. S., Goldsmith, M. and Goldsmith, P. (2018). Zika Virus: Patient Education Recommendations. *Adv Neonatal Care*, 18 (5): 360-365.

[197] Oster, A. M., Brooks, J. T., Stryker, J. E., Kachur, R. E., Mead, P., Pesik, N. T. and Petersen, L. R. (2016). Interim Guidelines for Prevention of Sexual Transmission of Zika Virus – United States, 2016. *MMWR Morb Mortal Wkly Rep*, 65 (5): 120-121.

[198] CDC Zika Response. (2016). Vital Signs: Preparing for Local Mosquito-Borne Transmission of Zika Virus – United States, 2016. *MMWR Morb Mortal Wkly Rep*, 65 (13): 352.

[199] Zika Working Group; Committee to Advise on Tropical Medicine; Travel (CATMAT). (2016). Canadian recommendations on the prevention and treatment of Zika virus: Update. *Can Commun Dis Rep*, 42 (5): 101-111.

[200] Mekala, H. M., Jayakumar, P., Yeruva, R. R. and Lippmann, S. (2016). What can we do about the Zika virus in the United States? *J Fam Pract*, 65 (11): 756-757.

[201] Wylie, B. J., Hauptman, M., Woolf, A. D. and Goldman, R. H. (2016). Insect Repellants during Pregnancy in the Era of the Zika Virus. *Obstet Gynecol*, 128 (5): 1111-1115.

[202] Hills, S. L., Russell, K., Hennessey, M., Williams, C., Oster, A. M., Fischer, M. and Mead, P. (2016). Transmission of Zika Virus through Sexual Contact with Travelers to Areas of Ongoing Transmission – Continental United States, 2016. *MMWR Morb Mortal Wkly Rep*, 65 (8): 215-216.

[203] Oster, A. M., Russell, K., Stryker, J. E., Friedman, A., Kachur, R. E., Petersen, E. E., Jamieson, D. J., Cohn, A. C. and Brooks, J. T. (2016). Update: Interim Guidance for Prevention of Sexual Transmission of Zika Virus – United States, 2016. *MMWR Morb Mortal Wkly Rep*, 65 (12): 323-325.

[204] Brooks, J. T., Friedman, A., Kachur, R. E., LaFlam, M., Peters, P. J. and Jamieson, D. J. (2016). Update: Interim Guidance for Prevention of Sexual Transmission of Zika Virus – United States, July 2016. *MMWR Morb Mortal Wkly Rep*, 65 (29): 745-747.

[205] Petersen, E. E., Meaney-Delman, D., Neblett-Fanfair, R., Havers, F., Oduyebo, T., Hills, S. L., Rabe, I. B., Lambert, A., Abercrombie, J., Martin, S. W., Gould, C. V., Oussayef, N., Polen, K. N., Kuehnert, M. J., Pillai, S. K., Petersen, L. R., Honein, M. A., Jamieson, D. J. and Brooks, J. T. (2016). Update: Interim Guidance for Preconception Counseling and Prevention of Sexual Transmission of Zika Virus for Persons with Possible Zika Virus Exposure – United States, September 2016. *MMWR Morb Mortal Wkly Rep*, 65 (39): 1077-1081.

[206] Polen, K. D., Gilboa, S. M., Hills, S., Oduyebo, T., Kohl, K. S., Brooks, J. T., Adamski, A., Simeone, R. M., Walker, A. T., Kissin, D. M., Petersen, L. R., Honein, M. A. and Meaney-Delman, D. (2018). Update: Interim Guidance for Preconception Counseling and Prevention of Sexual Transmission of Zika Virus for Men with Possible Zika Virus Exposure – United States, August 2018. *MMWR Morb Mortal Wkly Rep*, 67 (31): 868-871.

[207] Nguyen, B. T. and Schickler, R. (2018). Of mosquitoes and men: mitigating Zika risk via Men's family planning and male contraception. *Contracept Reprod Med*, 3: 17.

[208] Goldthwaite, L. M. and Velasquez, G. (2016). Family planning and the Zika era. *Curr Opin Obstet Gynecol*, 28 (6): 499-503.

[209] Dehlendorf, C., Gavin, L., Witt, J. and Moskosky, S. (2017). Facilitating State-Wide Collaboration around Family Planning Care in the Context of Zika. *Womens Health Issues*, 27 (4): 392-399.

[210] Maynard, A. D., Bowman, D. M. and Hodge, J. G. Jr. (2016). Mitigating Risks to Pregnant Teens from Zika Virus. *J Law Med Ethics*, 44 (4): 657-659.

[211] Schuck-Paim, C., López, D., Simonsen, L. and Alonso, W. (2016). Unintended Pregnancies in Brazil – A Challenge for the Recommendation to Delay Pregnancy Due to Zika. *PLoS Curr*, 8: pii.

[212] Darney, B. G., Aiken, A. R. and Küng, S. (2017). Access to Contraception in the Context of Zika: Health System Challenges and Responses. *Obstet Gynecol*, 129 (4): 638-642.

[213] Martinez, M. E. (2016). Preventing Zika Virus Infection during Pregnancy Using a Seasonal Window of Opportunity for Conception. *PLoS Biol*, 14 (7): e1002520.

[214] Ndeffo-Mbah, M. L., Parpia, A. S. and Galvani, A. P. (2016). Mitigating Prenatal Zika Virus Infection in the Americas. *Ann Intern Med*, 165 (8): 551-559.

[215] Tepper, N. K., Goldberg, H. I., Bernal, M. I., Rivera, B., Frey, M. T., Malave, C., Renquist, C. M., Bracero, N. J., Dominguez, K. L., Sanchez, R. E., Shapiro-Mendoza, C. K., Rodriguez, B. R., Simeone, R. M., Pesik, N. T., Barfield, W. D., Ko, J. Y., Galang, R. R., Perez-Padilla, J., Polen, K. N., Honein, M. A., Rasmussen, S. A. and Jamieson, D. J. (2016). Estimating Contraceptive Needs and Increasing Access to Contraception in Response to the Zika Virus Disease Outbreak – Puerto Rico, 2016. *MMWR Morb Mortal Wkly Rep*, 65 (12): 311-314.

[216] D'Angelo, D. V., Salvesen von Essen, B., Lamias, M. J., Shulman, H., Hernandez-Virella, W. I., Taraporewalla, A. J., Vargas, M. I., Harrison, L., Ellington, S. R., Soto, L., Williams, T., Rodriguez, A., Shapiro-Mendoza, C. K., Rivera, B., Cox, S., Pazol, K., Rice, M. E.,

Dee, D. L., Romero, L., Lathrop, E., Barfield, W., Smith, R. A., Jamieson, D. J., Honein, M. A., Deseda, C. and Warner, L. (2017). Measures Taken to Prevent Zika Virus Infection during Pregnancy – Puerto Rico, 2016. *MMWR Morb Mortal Wkly Rep*, 66 (22): 574-578.

[217] Prue, C. E., Roth, J. N. Jr., Garcia-Williams, A., Yoos, A., Camperlengo, L., DeWilde, L., Lamtahri, M., Prosper, A., Harrison, C., Witbart, L., Guendel, I., Wiegand, D. M., Lamens, N. R., Hillman, B., Davis, M. S. and Ellis, E. M. (2017). Awareness, Beliefs, and Actions Concerning Zika Virus Among Pregnant Women and Community Members – U.S. Virgin Islands, November-December 2016. *MMWR Morb Mortal Wkly Rep*, 66 (34): 909-913.

[218] Boulet, S. L., D'Angelo, D. V., Morrow, B., Zapata, L., Berry-Bibee, E., Rivera, M., Ellington, S., Romero, L., Lathrop, E., Frey, M., Williams, T., Goldberg, H., Warner, L., Harrison, L., Cox, S., Pazol, K., Barfield, W., Jamieson, D. J., Honein, M. A. and Kroelinger, C. D. (2016). Contraceptive Use among Nonpregnant and Postpartum Women at Risk for Unintended Pregnancy, and Female High School Students, in the Context of Zika Preparedness – United States, 2011-2013 and 2015. *MMWR Morb Mortal Wkly Rep*, 65 (30): 780-787.

[219] Burke, A. and Moreau, C. (2016). Family Planning and Zika Virus: The Power of Prevention. *Semin Reprod Med*, 34 (5): 305-312.

[220] Kroelinger, C. D., Romero, L., Lathrop, E., Cox, S., Morgan, I., Frey, M. T., Warner, L., Curtis, K. M., Pazol, K., Barfield, W. D., Meaney-Delman, D. and Jamieson, D. J. (2017). Meeting Summary: State and Local Implementation Strategies for Increasing Access to Contraception during Zika Preparedness and Response – United States, September 2016. *MMWR Morb Mortal Wkly Rep*, 66 (44): 1230-1235.

[221] Pazol, K., Ellington, S. R., Fulton, A. C., Zapata, L. B., Boulet, S. L., Rice, M. E., Cox, S., Romero, L., Lathrop, E., Hurst, S., Kroelinger, C. D., Goldberg, H., Shapiro-Mendoza, C. K., Simeone, R. M., Warner, L., Meaney-Delman, D. M. and Barfield, W. D.; Behavioral Risk Factor Surveillance System Family Planning Module Working

Group. (2018). Contraceptive Use among Women at Risk for Unintended Pregnancy in the Context of Public Health Emergencies – United States, 2016. *MMWR Morb Mortal Wkly Rep*, 67 (32): 898-902.

[222] Olson, C. K., Iwamoto, M., Perkins, K. M., Polen, K. N., Hageman, J., Meaney-Delman, D., Igbinosa, I. I., Khan, S., Honein, M. A., Bell, M., Rasmussen, S. A. and Jamieson, D. J. (2016). Preventing Transmission of Zika Virus in Labor and Delivery Settings through Implementation of Standard Precautions – United States, 2016. *MMWR Morb Mortal Wkly Rep*, 65 (11): 290-292.

[223] Goodnough, L. T. and Marques, M. B. (2017). Zika Virus and Patient Blood Management. *Anesth Analg*, 124 (1): 282-289.

[224] Kleinman, S. (2015). Pathogen inactivation: emerging indications. *Curr Opin Hematol*, 22 (6): 547-553.

[225] Pfaender, S., Vielle, N. J., Ebert, N., Steinmann, E., Alves, M. P. and Thiel, V. (2017). Inactivation of Zika virus in human breast milk by prolonged storage or pasteurization. *Virus Res*, 228: 58-60.

[226] Dawes, B. E., Smalley, C. A., Tiner, B. L., Beasley, D. W., Milligan, G. N., Reece, L. M., Hombach, J. and Barrett, A. D. (2016). Research and development of Zika virus vaccines. *NPJ Vaccines*, 1: 16007.

[227] Monath, T. P., Craven, R. B., Muth, D. J., Trautt, C. J., Calisher, C. H. and Fitzgerald, S. A. (1980). Limitations of the complement-fixation test for distinguishing naturally acquired from vaccine-induced yellow fever infection in flavivirus-hyperendemic areas. *Am J Trop Med Hyg*, 29 (4): 624-634.

[228] Vouga, M., Alves, M. P., Eperon, I., Eperon, G., Rochat, L., Sahli, R., Musso, D. and Baud, D. (2016). Zika virus: from research to vaccine. *Rev Med Suisse*, 12 (536): 1794-1798.

[229] Singh, M. V., Weber, E. A., Singh, V. B., Stirpe, N. E. and Maggirwar, S. B. (2017). Preventive and therapeutic challenges in combating Zika virus infection: are we getting any closer? *J Neurovirol*, 23 (3): 347-357.

[230] Martinez-Palomo, A. (2016). Revisiting Zika (and Rubella). *J Public Health Policy*, 37 (3): 273-276.

[231] Durbin, A. P. (2016). Vaccine Development for Zika Virus – Timelines and Strategies. *Semin Reprod Med*, 34 (5): 299-304.

[232] Heinz, F. X. and Stiasny, K. (2017). The Antigenic Structure of Zika Virus and Its Relation to Other Flaviviruses: Implications for Infection and Immunoprophylaxis. *Microbiol Mol Biol Rev*, 81 (1): e00055-16.

[233] Rather, I. A., Kumar, S., Bajpai, V. K., Lim, J. and Park, Y. H. (2017). Prevention and Control Strategies to Counter ZIKA Epidemic. *Front Microbiol*, 8: 305.

[234] Eperon, G., Schibler, M., Wagner, N., Chappuis, F. and Eperon, I. (2017). Zika virus: practical guidelines. *Rev Med Suisse*, 13 (561): 938-943.

[235] McArthur, M. A. (2017). Zika Virus: Recent Advances towards the Development of Vaccines and Therapeutics. *Viruses*, 9 (6): E143.

[236] Lagunas-Rangel, F. A., Viveros-Sandoval, M. E. and Reyes-Sandoval, A. (2017). Current trends in Zika vaccine development. *J Virus Erad*, 3 (3): 124-127.

[237] Durbin, A. and Wilder-Smith, A. (2017). An update on Zika vaccine developments. *Expert Rev Vaccines*, 16 (8): 781-787.

[238] Wahid, B., Ali, A., Rafique, S. and Idrees, M. (2017). Current status of therapeutic and vaccine approaches against Zika virus. *Eur J Intern Med*, 44: 12-18.

[239] Stein, D. R., Golden, J. W., Griffin, B. D., Warner, B. M., Ranadheera, C., Scharikow, L., Sloan, A., Frost, K. L., Kobasa, D., Booth, S. A., Josleyn, M., Ballantyne, J., Sullivan, E., Jiao, J. A., Wu, H., Wang, Z., Hooper, J. W. and Safronetz, D. (2017). Human polyclonal antibodies produced in transchromosomal cattle prevent lethal Zika virus infection and testicular atrophy in mice. *Antiviral Res*, 146: 164-173.

[240] Schwartz, D. A. (2018). Clinical Trials and Administration of Zika Virus Vaccine in Pregnant Women: Lessons (that Should Have Been) Learned from Excluding Immunization with the Ebola

Vaccine during Pregnancy and Lactation. *Vaccines (Basel)*, 6 (4): E81.

[241] Valega-Mackenzie, W. and Ríos-Soto, K. R. (2018). Can Vaccination Save a Zika Virus Epidemic? *Bull Math Biol*, 80 (3): 598-625.

[242] Masmejan, S., Baud, D., Musso, D. and Panchaud, A. (2018). Zika virus, vaccines, and antiviral strategies. *Expert Rev Anti Infect Ther*, 16 (6): 471-483.

[243] Shan, C., Xie, X. and Shi, P. Y. (2018). Zika Virus Vaccine: Progress and Challenges. *Cell Host Microbe*, 24 (1): 12-17.

[244] Diamond, M. S., Ledgerwood, J. E. and Pierson, T. C. (2019). Zika Virus Vaccine Development: Progress in the Face of New Challenges. *Annu Rev Med*, 70: 121-135.

[245] Sinigaglia, A., Riccetti, S., Trevisan, M. and Barzon, L. (2018). In silico approaches to Zika virus drug discovery. *Expert Opin Drug Discov*, 13 (9): 825-835.

[246] Salam, A. P., Rojek, A., Dunning, J. and Horby, P. W. (2017). Clinical Trials of Therapeutics for the Prevention of Congenital Zika Virus Disease: Challenges and Potential Solutions. *Ann Intern Med*, 166 (10): 725-732.

[247] Munjal, A., Khandia, R., Dhama, K., Sachan, S., Karthik, K., Tiwari, R., Malik, Y. S., Kumar, D., Singh, R. K., Iqbal, H. M. N. and Joshi, S. K. (2017). Advances in Developing Therapies to Combat Zika Virus: Current Knowledge and Future Perspectives. *Front Microbiol*, 8: 1469.

[248] Hall, R. A. and Macdonald, J. (2016). Synthetic Biology Provides a Toehold in the Fight against Zika. *Cell Host Microbe*, 19 (6): 752-754.

[249] De Moraes Gomes, P. A. T., Pena, L. J. and Leite, A. C. L. (2019). Isatin Derivatives and Their Antiviral Properties against Arboviruses: A Review. *Mini Rev Med Chem*, 19 (1): 56-62.

[250] Sukhralia, S., Verma, M., Gopirajan, S., Dhanaraj, P. S., Lal, R., Mehla, N. and Kant, C. R. (2019). From dengue to Zika: the wide

spread of mosquito-borne arboviruses. *Eur J Clin Microbiol Infect Dis*, 38 (1): 3-14.

[251] Alvarado, M. G. and Schwartz, D. A. (2017). Zika Virus Infection in Pregnancy, Microcephaly, and Maternal and Fetal Health: What We Think, What We Know, and What We Think We Know. *Arch Pathol Lab Med*, 141 (1): 26-32.

[252] Arnaoutakis, D. and Padhya, T. (2017). Zika Virus – What the Otolaryngologist Should Know: A Review. *JAMA Otolaryngol Head Neck Surg*, 143 (1): 81-84.

[253] Soriano-Arandes, A., Rivero-Calle, I., Nastouli, E., Espiau, M., Frick, M. A., Alarcon, A. and Martinón-Torres, F. (2018). What we know and what we don't know about perinatal Zika virus infection: a systematic review. *Expert Rev Anti Infect Ther*, 16 (3): 243-254.

In: Advances in Health and Disease
Editor: Lowell T. Duncan
ISBN: 978-1-53616-380-3

Chapter 2

MULTIPLE MYELOMA: BIOLOGICAL CHARACTERISTICS, CLINICAL ASPECTS AND THERAPEUTIC APPROACHES

***Sara Grammatico*[1,*]**
***and Maria Teresa Petrucci*[2]**
[1]Clinical Hematology and Oncohematology,
Hospital of Prato "Santo Stefano", Prato, Italy
[2]Hematology, Azienda Policlinico Umberto I,
"Sapienza" University, Rome, Italy

ABSTRACT

Multiple myeloma is characterized by the expansion of monoclonal plasma cells in the bone marrow. In about 95% of cases the aberrant plasma cells produce a monoclonal immunoglobulin called monoclonal component that can be considered a marker of the disease. Multiple myeloma diagnostic criteria include: bone marrow plasmacytosis, the presence of monoclonal protein in the serum and/or urine and the

[*]Corresponding Author's Email: sara.grammatico@uslcentro.toscana.it.

presence of one of these signs and symptoms, the so-called CRAB manifestation: hypercalcemia (C), renal insufficiency (R), bone marrow insufficiency (especially anemia) (A) and/or osteolytic lesions (B). The more recent revision of these criteria allows the diagnosis of multiple myeloma even in absence of the CRAB manifestation, if one of these condition is present: >60% of plasma cells in the bone marrow, a value of serum Free Light Chains ratio>100, or>1 focal lesion identified by magnetic resonance.

Over the last few decades, the introduction of intensive treatments, such as high dose chemotherapy followed by autologous stem cell transplantation and novel agents, including immunomodulatory drugs (thalidomide, lenalidomide and pomalidomide), proteosome inhibitors (bortezomib, carfilzomib, ixazomib), and monoclonal antibodies (elotuzumab and daratumumab), has markedly improved the outcome of multiple myeloma patients. Three-drugs combinations, including at least bortezomib or lenalidomide, are now routinely used as induction therapy for young newly diagnosed patients, followed by high-dose chemotherapy and autologous transplantation. Bortezomib and lenalidomide are also commonly used as induction therapy for elderly patients within different regimens.

Treatment for relapse/refractory patients includes combinations of new-generation agents (such as carfilzomib, ixazomib, elotuzumab and daratumumab with lenalidomide and dexamethasone or daratumumab with bortezomib and dexamethasone) but also monotherapy (pomalidomide or daratumumab).

A deep knowledge of the toxicities of all these novel drugs is mandatory to better manage all potential side effects and to reduce the risk of treatment discontinuation or serious adverse events.

Given the wide range of therapeutic regimens that are now available, the choice of the best treatment cannot be so obvious. Therefore, it must be necessary to draw homogeneous therapeutic guidelines to identify the best sequence of treatment to adopt during the course of the disease and also the precise timing (at biochemical relapse or clinical relapse).

Moreover, a deeper characterization of patients (by phenotype, cytogenetic and molecular biology) and the evaluation of minimal residual disease would guide the choice in the treatment of multiple myeloma patients.

INTRODUCTION

Multiple myeloma (MM) is a malignant tumour of the hematopoietic system that falls into a heterogeneous group of diseases called plasma cells dyscrasias, characterized by the expansion of monoclonal plasma cells in the bone marrow. In about 95% of cases that disease produces a monoclonal immunoglobulin called paraprotein or monoclonal component (M-protein). Such paraprotein in serum and/or urine generally migrates to position γ at the electrophoretic pathway and can be considered as a marker of such disease. Myeloma proteins have an altered structure due to mutations in immunoglobulin genes; sometimes the molecule breaks down and myeloma cells produce only light chains (Bence Jones proteinuria), or only heavy chains (causing a rare condition as "heavy chain disease") or eventually molecular fragments. In general, the distribution of monoclonal gammopathies depending on the type of immunoglobulin involved: IgGs are the most common ones, affecting 70% of cases, followed by IgM in 15% and IgA in 12%; rare are light chain and biclonal or IgD and IgE [1].

Usually the paraprotein is defective, resulting in loss of normal antibody function. MM therefore represents an altered immune response characterized by the proliferation of neoplastic cells with suppression of normal plasmocytes and this result in lowering normal immunoglobulin levels.

In rare cases (<1%), myeloma cells do not produce any immunoglobulin and therefore it is called non-secretory myeloma without evidence of paraprotein neither in the serum nor in the urine. Sometimes plasma cells can proliferate also extramedullary, providing the so-called plasmacytoma. However, in some cases, plasma cells proliferation is located only at one extramedullary localization or in a single tissue outside the bone, without the bone marrow involvement, leading to the solitary bone plasmacytoma or solitary extramedullary plasmacytoma, respectively.

Despite the fact that MM is characterized by the M-protein, the paraprotein is not always synonymous of neoplasia. In fact, it is important to differentiate patients with malignant conditions such as symptomatic myeloma, solitary plasmacytoma and plasma cell leukemia, which need to be treated immediately, and benign forms such as monoclonal gammopathies of undetermined significance (MGUS) and smouldering multiple myeloma (SMM), which need just observation to assess the possible evolution of the disease. The distinction is very important considering the different clinical and therapeutic approaches that these different entities need.

Recently, Kyle et al. Evaluated a large group of 1384 patients with MGUS: 11% have progression. The risk of progression without accounting for death due to competing causes was 10% at 10 years, 18% at 20 years, 28% at 30 years, 36% at 35 years, and 36% at 40 years. Adverse risk factors for progression are an abnormal Free Light Chain ratio (FLCr) and a high M-protein level [1].

Also for SMM there are adverse risk factors for progression such as bone marrow plasma cells > 20%, M-protein > 2 g/dL, and FLCr > 20 at diagnosis [2].

Nowadays, there are some clinical trials that evaluate the role of new agents, for example lenalidomide, carfilzomib or monoclonal antibodies as elotuzumab or daratumumab, for the treatment of SMM, especially for high risks patients [3-5]. These trials provide good results in terms of percentage of evolution in MM; however, outside the clinical trials, the approach in the real practice for SMM, is still observation.

EPIDEMIOLOGY

MM can be considered a tumour of the elderly, affecting in 50% of cases patients older than 60-65 years with a male/female ratio of 3: 2. The median age at diagnosis is 69 years; 28.6% of patients are aged between 65 and 74 years, and 33% are older than 75 years. Only 14% of patients are diagnosed while younger than 55 years [6].

Its incidence in the world is very variable, ranging from the Chinese minimum of 1/100,000 to about 4/100,000 in most industrialized western countries. However, the improving diagnostic techniques and the increasing average age of the population could explain in part the raise in its incidence recorded in recent decades. The tendency for increased frequency in patients with less than 55 years of age over the past 3-4 decades, reporting cases in patients under 30-35 years old, underlines the possible greater importance of environmental factors in triggering the disease.

Ethyopathogenesis

The etiology of MM is largely unknown, although it is possible to suggest the role of some genetic factors (some studies have suggested an association between MM and certain histocompatibility antigens such as B5, CW5 and CW2), environmental (radiation, toxic agents) and some pathological conditions (infections, autoimmune or dysmetabolic diseases) in the pathogenesis of the disease.

Biology

From the morphological and functional point of view, the tumour cell responsible of MM is the plasma cell, the mature cell of B lymphocyte, that is incapable of supporting tumour proliferation. Numerous studies have suggested an involvement of more immature B cells than plasma cells, also present in peripheral blood [7, 8].

This hypothesis is supported by data relating to the phenotype [9].

Pre-B cell expansion is considered to be a crucial step in the pathogenesis of MM, with the addition of genetic alterations that cause the development of the disease.

Cytokines

Another controversy, not yet clarified, is the role of interleukin-6 (IL-6), which is considered to be the most important growth factor for the development of MM. Although initial studies suggest that this cytokine is self-produced by plasma cells [10], other researchers support paracrine production of this molecule that stimulate the growth of plasma cells [11]. In addition, the expression and production of IL-6 by less mature cells has been clearly demonstrated [12] by evaluating IL-6 gene expression in purified plasma cells. More mature cells lose expression of IL-6 and hence the ability to respond to this cytokine, as also demonstrated by the loss of IL-6 receptor expression. This cytokine can promote neoplastic proliferation, but also make the myeloma cells resistant to the action of certain drugs such as cortisone, interfering with the mechanisms that control the phenomenon of apoptosis [13]. IL-6 also plays a key role in the pathogenesis of osteolytic lesions; in fact, together with its soluble receptor and IL1-α induces the activation of osteoclasts by causing bone resorption [14]. Along with IL-6 to mention are other cytokines such as the granulocyte-colony stimulating factor (G-CSF), interferon alfa (IFN-α) and IL-11 that exert their action through the same IL receptor -6. The role of IL-10 has also been reported, which is another cytokine able to stimulate plasma cells proliferation.

Osteolytic lesions of MM are the product of an imbalance between bone formation by osteoblasts and destruction by osteoclasts. The increase in osteoclast activity observed in MM patients is due to an imbalance between the receptor activator of nuclear factor kB (RANK) and osteoprotegerin (OPG) due in turn to an increase in production of RANK ligand (RANKL) and a reduced production of osteoprotegerin. Stromal damage is so important that bone reconstruction is rarely observed even in patients with complete remission [15].

CYTOGENETICS

The mitotic activity of plasma cells in MM is higher than that in normal subjects and varies depending on the state of the disease. It is certainly higher in patients with a resistant disease than those at onset of disease, but it is far less than that of other neoplastic diseases. However, despite the difficulties of this low proliferative activity, cytogenetic studies have demonstrated the presence of karyotype alterations in 40% of cases, with a lower frequency in diagnosed patients than those evaluated at advanced disease.

Some chromosomal regions are frequently involved in these aberrations, revealing the role of some oncogenes in the pathogenesis of MM. Among these oncogenes, an important role is attributable to the altered regulation of proteins such as ras, bcl-2 and c- Myc and the loss of protein products of suppressor genes such as retinoblastoma and p53, which are the basis of molecular mechanisms that induce resistance to drugs and radiation in MM.

Primary and secondary genetic abnormalities (predominantly translocations) are recognized. Primary translocations involve 40-50% of patients in the 14q32 region (IgH) of immunoglobulins and are common to MM and MGUS [16]. These injuries are therefore indispensable to the development of gammopathy, while a second ("second hit") is required for neoplastic evolution. Thus, secondary lesions appear with the progression of the disease and include loss of chromosome 13, NRAS and KRAS oncogenes activating mutations, inactivating mutations or deletions of p53, PTEN inactivation [17, 18].

Patients with MM may be subdivided into groups that exhibit hyperdiploid and non hyperdiploid plasma cells clones. Based on hyper- or hypodiploids and chromosomal translocations involving the 14q32 region, different subgroups of patients with different prognoses can be identified [19]. The chromosomal/genomic characteristics of patients can therefore be used as prognostic parameters. However, to date the chromosomal characterization of the disease does not correspond to a specific standardized therapeutic approach.

According to the International Myeloma Working Group (IMWG), deletion of the chromosome 17, translocation t(4;14)(p16;q32), translocation t(14;16)(q32;q23), translocation t(14;20)(q32;q11), deletion or gain of chromosome 1, deletion of chromosome 13 are considered at high risks [20].

PHENOTYPE

The use of monoclonal antibodies allows identifying the phenotype of tumour cells from normal plasma cells. Myeloma plasma cells show a significant antigenic heterogeneity, also due to the different antibody expression that varies in relation to the maturation status of pathological plasma cells. The strong expression of the CD38 antigen allows the distinction of plasma cells from other hemopoietic cells, while the distinction between normal and pathological would be based on the study of other antigens such as VLA4, VLA5, MPC1, CD44, but especially CD19 which is positive in normal plasma cells while CD56, CD20, CD24 and CD10 are negative. Although it has not yet clearly demonstrated the role of the CD56, this antigen, in association with CD19 expression, makes it possible to clearly distinguish pathological plasma cells from the normal ones. The latter are CD56- and CD19+, and the most mature in the majority are CD56+ and CD19- and a small minority of CD56- CD19- and CD56+ and CD19+. More recently, another antigen, CD138 (syndecan-1) has been identified on the surface of myeloma plasma cells; this antigen, which is part of the adhesion molecule group, promotes and maintains the aggregation of myeloma cells at the bone marrow level, while it is lost by the plasma cells that are found in peripheral blood in the case of plasma cell leukaemia.

The probability of detecting probable specific antigens of this disease by flow cytometry could be particularly useful in evaluating the minimum residual disease (MRD).

PROGNOSTIC FACTORS

Prognosis depends on either the number of neoplastic cells or specific characteristics of the disease, including β2-microglobulin, protein C reactive (CRP), serum creatinine and patient age at diagnosis.

B2-microglobulin, which is the light chain component of classical HLA antigens present on the surface of cells, is a low molecular weight protein (11,800 dalton). It can be increased in the serum and urine of patients with inflammatory and malignant diseases. In MM patients its serum levels correlate with tumour mass when evaluated prior to therapy. Furthermore, it has been shown that high levels of β2-microglobulin are associated with a significantly reduced survival and that its measurement can provide information similar to those obtained from M-protein levels in seriated monitoring of such patients.

CRP is directly related to the activity of IL-6, which, as mentioned, is the most important growth factor of the plasma cells. High CPR values are often present in the serum of patients undergoing diagnosis and during recovery of the disease, while they are low in the remission phase.

Serum creatinine is a very important parameter of renal function evaluation, which is particularly important for MM patients, considering the frequent impairment of the organ.

The age of the patient to diagnosis is another prognostic factor that plays a key role in the therapeutic choice.

As mentioned above, also cytogenetic aberrations play an important prognostic role.

STAGING

Despite the numerous attempts to evaluate parameters that are able to classify this tumour differently, the Durie and Salmon system reported in 1975 still remains valid [21]. This system correlates the most important clinical parameters (paraprotein, hemoglobin and calcium, presence of osteolytic lesions) with the cellular mass of this neoplasia (Figure 1).

Subsequently, Greipp [22] presented a new stage system which, however, did not replace the old classification, and is based on two parameters: β2-microglobulin (cut-off 4 μg/ml) and plasma cell labeling indices (cut-off 0.4%). Patients according to the values of these two parameters are divided into three stages: low, intermediate and high risk.

- **STAGE I – median survival 60 months**
  - **Hemoglobin > 10 g/dl**
  - **Calcium normal**
  - **One lytic lesion at skeleton survey**
  - **M-protein: IgG < 5 g/dl; IgA < 3 g/dl; BJ proteinuria < 4 gr/24 hr.**
- **STAGE II – median survival 40 months**
  - **Intermediate**
- **STAGE III – median survival 20 months**
  - **Hemoglobin < 8,5 g/dl**
  - **Calcium > 12 mg/ml**
  - **More than one lytic lesion**
  - **M-protein: IgG > 7 g/dl; IgA > 5 g/dl; BJ proteinuria > 12 gr/24 hr**
- **Subgroups:**
  - **A: creatinine <2.0 mg/dl**
  - **B : creatinine >2.0 mg/dl**

Figure 1. Durie and Salmon staging system. BJ: Bence Jones proteinuria; g/dl: gram/deciliter; mg/dl: milligram/deciliter.

In 1992 Battaille proposed another staging by dividing patients relative to β2-microglobulin and CRP values. Using an identical cut-off for the two parameters (6 mg/l), according to this classification, patients are divided into three risk groups: low, intermediate and high [23].

Numerous other prognostic factors are considered, including molecular alterations such as oncogenic and anti-oncogenic mutations, which, however, require very expensive examinations such as FISH; thus these alterations are still not routinely used in clinical practice outside experimental trials.

The International Staging System (ISS) is a more cost-effective alternative to the Durie-Salmon staging system [24]. The ISS is based on the assessment of two blood test results: beta 2-microglobulin and albumin. This evaluation has shown the greatest prognostic power for MM, and it has already been proven more sensitive in discriminating between three stages of myeloma. These stages indicate different levels of projected survival rates.

More recently, the Revised International Staging System (RISS) has combined elements of tumour burden (ISS) and disease biology (presence of high-risk cytogenetic abnormalities or elevated lactate dehydrogenase level) to create a unified prognostic index that helps in clinical care as well as in comparison of clinical trial data [25].

DIAGNOSIS

The suspected diagnosis of MM is always present in the presence of an alteration of the serum and/or urine protein framework, which in 90% of cases is randomly detected during routine investigations that increasingly include the study of protein electrophoresis. In the presence of such an alteration, laboratory and instrumental examinations will be required to distinguish the various types of plasma cell dyscrasia and to evaluate the need for any treatment (Figure 2).

✓ Clinical history and physical examination

✓ Complete blood count with formula

✓Chemistry (calcium, creatinine, CRP, β2microglobuline, dosage Ig, FLC)

✓ EF serum with IFX

✓ BJ urine of 24h

✓ Bone marrow aspirate (with immunophenotype and cytogenetic analysis)

✓ Imaging studies of the skeleton (X-ray, CT, MRI and/or PET)

Figure 2. Diagnostic work-up for MM. CRP: protein C reactive; Ig: immunoglobulins; FLC: free light chain; EF: electrophoresis; IFX: immunofixation; BJ: Bence Jones proteinuria, CT: computed tomography; MRI: magnetic resonance imaging; PET:18 Fluorodeoxyglucose positron emission tomography.

The complete blood count examination allows evaluating anemia, that is usually macrocytic, and other possible peripheral cytopenias. The quantitative and qualitative study of serum M-protein and/or Bence Jones proteinuria are evaluated by electrophoresis, immunofixation and the dosage of serum and urinary immunoglobulins. Biochemical examinations including calcium, creatinine, albumin, β2-microglobulin and PCR assays allow the evaluation of serum calcium levels, renal function and disease activity. In addition, the free light chains (FLCs) assay, that provides quantitation of kappa and lambda chains not bound to intact immunoglobulin molecules and allows the determination of clonality based on the FLCr, can define more precisely the diagnosis of MM (involved:uninvolved serum FLCr§ ≥100) [26].

Bone marrow aspiration, with morphologic, immunophenotypic and cytogenetic analysis is essential for diagnosis of MM. Bone marrow biopsy is mandatory in case of non-secretory MM (without evidence of M-protein in serum or urine) and in case of solitary plasmacytoma to exclude the bone marrow involvement. The presence of monoclonal plasma cells can be accurately evaluated by cytofluorimetry using anti-CD138 antibodies. In addition, preferably on purified plasma cells, the "fluorescent in situ hybridization" (FISH) with probes including the del17p13, t(4; 14), t(14; 16); t(14;20) and chromosome 1 lead to the identification of chromosomal aberrations that can have prognostic implications [27].

Possible bone lesions are evaluated with radiological examinations such as, at least standard radiographs of the entire skeleton and/or computed tomography (CT), magnetic resonance imaging (MRI) or 18 Fluorodeoxyglucose positron emission tomography (FDG PET). Bone scintigraphy, is not recommended for the many false negatives due to the failure to activate osteoblasts in response to bone destruction by activated osteoclasts. In the case of negative radiographies, it may be necessary to carry out an MRI, which is also useful for highlighting not only bone marrow involvement but also possible spinal compression [28]. On the contrary, the FDG PET is very useful for the identification of extra-marrow disease, whereas, for the bone marrow study, MRI has shown greater sensitivity to the identification of bone myeloma lesions compared to FDG

PET. However, in recent years, great attention has been paid to the use of FDG PET for identifying predictive factors for long-term therapy and survival, similar to those occurring for other neoplastic diseases (eg lymphomas). Analysis of the metabolic activity of the disease by FDG PET has been shown to be a statistically significant prognostic factor both in diagnosis and in monitoring the response during therapy [29, 30]. An extended capture, high capture intensity (in terms of Standardized Uptake Value) and the presence of extra-marrow disease at the diagnosis are unfavourable prognostic elements. Concerning the evaluation of response to therapy, the signal suppression correlates with the biochemical response obtained after chemotherapy: the persistence of FDG PET positivity is significantly associated with a lower survival than patients in whom FDG PET is found to be negative.

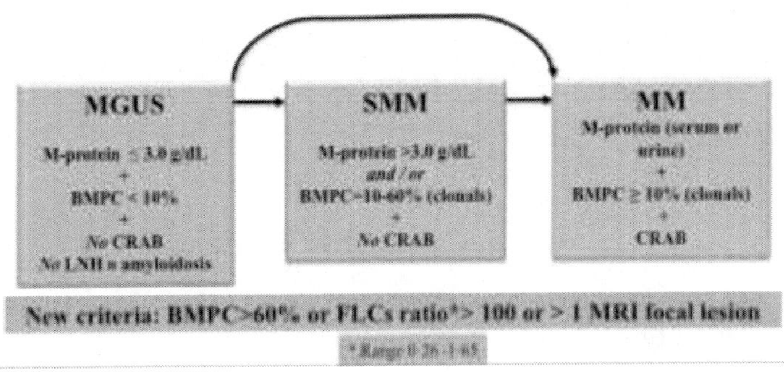

Figure 3. Diagnostic criteria for MM. MGUS: monoclonal gammopathies of undetermined significance; SMM: smouldering multiple myeloma; MM: multiple myeloma; BMPC: bone marrow plasma cells; FLCs: free light chains; MRI: magnetic resonance imaging.

The classic criteria for diagnosis of MM are based on the presence of bone marrow plasmacytosis, the presence of M-protein or the presence of signs and symptoms, the so-called CRAB manifestation (hypercalcemia, renal insufficiency, anemia and/or bone lesions). SMM is considered an asymptomatic MM; however, some studies reported specific cases of SMM with a very high risk of development into symptomatic MM [31]. Therefore, in 2014, new MM diagnostic criteria had been developed by the IMWG, extending the diagnosis of active MM also to forms of SMM at high risk of progression (>60% of plasma cells bone marrow invasion, Serum FLCr> 100,> 1 focal lesion identified by MRI) (Figure 3).

According to the new criteria, it is possible to define:

- MGUS: IgG or IgA monoclonal component <3 g/dl (<0.5 g/day if urinary component) with a bone marrow monoclonal plasma cells<10% and in the absence of symptoms;
- SMM: IgG or IgA monoclonal component ≥3 g/dl (≥0.5 g/dl if urinary component) or a 10-60% bone marrow monoclonal plasma cells count, without any symptoms;
- MM:
  - ≥10% of bone marrow monoclonal plasma cells or extra-marrow plasmacytoma and CRAB symptoms
  - >60% of bone marrow monoclonal plasma cells
  - FLCr> 100 mg/dl
  - >focal lesions highlighted by MRI.

Signs and Symptoms

CRAB symptoms:

- *Hypercalcemia:* directly related to bone remodeling. It may be symptomatic (anorexia, polyuria and polydipsia, up to squares of vomiting and dehydration nausea and ultimately signs of encephalopathy in severe cases) and may in some cases be aggravated by concomitant renal failure.
- *Renal insufficiency:* the pathogenesis is multifactorial, with a primary role played by the excess of light monoclonal chains in plasma, filtered at the glomerular level and then reabsorbed and catabolized at tubular level. During these processes, light chains may precipitate at intratubular level, depositing at the basal membrane of tubules or glomeruli or causing direct or mediated

cellular damage. The most frequent morphological and functional aspect is myeloma kidney, whose most common clinical manifestation is chronic kidney failure (an acute renal failure framework is rarer and generally occurs when other precipitating factors such as hyperuricemia, dehydration, etc.); less frequent light chain disease and amyloidosis.

- *Bone marrow insufficiency:* the inability to produce normal blood cells due to the proliferation of myeloma cells leading to the progressive replacement of normal cellular lineages. Paleos, asthenia, tachycardia, stress or rest disorder are symptoms that affect about 40% of patients who are just anemic. Anemia in many patients is also due to a hemodilution that is secondary to the presence and concentration of M-protein and yet to a possible endogenous erythropoietin production deficiency that may be related to renal impairment. Neutropenia and trombocytopenia are less common symptoms in these patients but associated with other factors such as reduced production of normal immunoglobulins and M-protein interference with coagulation factors, in some cases contributing to increased susceptibility to infections and hemorrhagic symptoms that are usually limited to the skin, but may also be due to mucous membranes and parenchymas.
- *Bone involvement:* severe osteoporosis or osteolytic lesions are often responsible for pathological fractures, spinal cord compression, hypercalcemia and bone pain. These lesions can affect any skeletal segment. Bone pains are often very severe and are the cause of an unacceptable quality of life. Bone destruction is related to increased bone resorption with reduction in the formation of new bone matrix. Excessive osteoclast activity is generally a very early process in this disease, while inhibition of osteoblast activity appears later.

In addition to the aforementioned hemodilution and hemorrhagic symptoms due to the interference with other plasma proteins such as coagulation factors (I, II, V, VII, VIII) and platelet membrane proteins, M-protein may be responsible of increased blood viscosity. This may be due to the physical characteristics of M-protein, which is more pronounced in myeloma IgA (dimer) and IgM (pentamerum) than IgG. Symptoms can vary from modest headaches and dizziness to a true hyperviscosity syndrome. The latter causes, at the microcirculation level, a slowing down of the flow with distension and tortuosity of vessels easily evaluable with the examination of the ocular fund. It may be cause congestive heart failure due to increased cardiac work as a result of increased flow resistance. Peripheral symptomatology is characterized by hemorrhagic syndrome and circulatory insufficiency especially in the lower limbs, while at the cerebral level there is reduction of visus due to retinal microhemorrhages and neurological symptoms such as headache, ear arousal, difficulty concentrating, drowsiness, degeneration of the sensory until to coma.

Finally, M-protein can directly cause functional damage by depositing itself in the various organs. This is particularly common in the kidneys at both tubule and glomerular levels, causing a progressive picture of chronic renal failure.

A particular picture due to the deposition of M-protein is secondary amyloidosis, which is due to a clinical picture very similar to primary amyloidosis and affects 10% of patients with MM. For its diagnosis it is indispensable to demonstrate the deposition of the amyloid substance in the various organs (subcutaneous tissue, intestinal mucosa, gums, etc.), highlighted with red congo coloration, of histological preparations which, when positive, give a typical green fluorescence with polarized light. The most typical sign of amyloidosis is organomegaly; typical, in fact, is the volumetric increase of the tongue, liver and heart, with the possibility of functional hepatic and cardiac deficiency. It is possible to have chronic renal failure due to kidney involvement, congestive heart failure and rhythm disturbances for heart failure, and still distal sensory neuropathies and malabsorption syndrome, respectively, for peripheral and intestinal nerves. Functional reduction of wrist and finger joint movements may occur in the case of carpal tunnel syndrome due to the deposition of M-protein.

Treatment Approaches

The outcome of MM patients has markedly improved over the past decade, both in young and elderly patients. In the past years, conventional therapy, such as melphalan plus prednisone (MP), was the only active treatment against MM. Since the 1980s, high doses of chemotherapy plus autologous stem cell transplantation (ASCT) proved to be the most suitable option for young newly diagnosed MM (YNDMM) patients [32, 33]. More recently, new active classes of drugs, such as proteasome inhibitors-PIs (e.g., bortezomib) and immunomodulatory drugs-IMiDs (e.g., thalidomide and lenalidomide) became the standard of care, alone or in association with the old agents, either for first-line therapy in the transplant and non-transplant settings, or for the treatment of relapsed disease.

In the setting of YNDMM patients, novel agents showed better responses than the old conventional drugs in numerous studies [34-36]. In the light of these results, nowadays, novel agents have become the standard treatment for these patients. Different combinations with novel agents as induction therapy for ASCT have been explored. Doublet therapies combining either an IMiD or bortezomib with dexamethasone (eg, thalidomide and dexamethasone-TD or lenalidomide and dexamethasone-Rd or bortezomib and dexamethasone-VD) affected higher overall response rates than traditional treatments [34, 35, 37-40]. However, triplet induction regimens, in particular, bortezomib plus thalidomide and dexamethasone (VTD), further increased the rate of complete remission (CR) and/or at least Very Good Partial Response (VGPR), both before and after ASCT [41-43].

Several newer induction treatments, such as bortezomib plus lenalidomide and dexamethasone (VRd), bortezomib plus cyclophos-phamide and dexamethasone (VCD), bortezomib plus doxorubicin, and dexamethasone (PAD) and Rd, have been also included as a category 1 recommendation in the United States National Comprehensive Cancer Network Clinical Practice Guidelines in Oncology for Multiple Myeloma Version 1.2011.23. [44-47, 36]. Four-drugs induction regimens have been also investigated, but toxicities appeared too high respect to a real advantage in terms of efficacy [48, 49].

In summary, latest 2015 IMWG recommendation provided the use of a three-drug regimen based on bortezomib/dexamethasone, with the addition of a third agent as cyclophosphamide, adriamycin, thalidomide, or lenalidomide [46].

In the absence of randomized studies comparing different induction regimens, it is difficult to recommend one induction regimen over another. However, biological and clinical characteristics of patients at the onset may influence the choice. For example, high-risk patients with t(4;14), translocation or deletion of chromosome 17p could benefit from bortezomib-based regimen. In the presence of patients with comorbidities, for example acute renal failure or thromboembolic disease, bortezomib-based regimens should be used, while patients with pre-existing neuropathy could be treated with lenalidomide-based regimens.

After induction treatment, consolidation with high-dose chemotherapy and ASCT still remains the standard care for YNDMM. Novel agents have also shown efficacy as maintenance treatment post-ASCT, even if only thalidomide and lenalidomide are actually allowed outside clinical trials.

In the era of novel agents, numerous issues arise. One is the length of induction treatment: the choice of giving 3 to 6 cycles of induction therapy depends on the depth of response and toxicity observed.

Another question is the number of transplants and the timing of transplantation. Some retrospective trials analysed the role of early versus delayed ASCT after novel agents and progression-free survival (PFS) and overall survival (OS) were similar [50, 51]. However, there are few prospective trials that compare novel agents versus ASCT; data seem to be in favour of ASCT [52, 53]. Palumbo et al. reported that ASCT, compared with melphalan, prednisone and lenalidomide (MPR) consolidation, significantly prolonged PFS and OS [54]. Therefore, until further clinical trials will definitively answer to this question, ASCT, performed after induction with novel agents, still remain the treatment of choice.

Autologous transplantation may be single or tandem (a planned second course of ASCT within 6 months of the first). Studies performed in the old era, showed improvement in OS with tandem ASCT [55]; this is confirmed particularly in patients who failed to achieve at least a VGPR [56, 57]. Also with novel agents, some groups strongly suggested tandem ASCT in case of MRD positivity after induction therapy. Moreover, recent studies suggest that there is a role for tandem ASCT in the presence of adverse cytogenetic abnormalities [58, 59].

Novel agents are also used as induction therapy for elderly patients not eligible for ASCT. Combinations of melphalan, prednisone with thalidomide (MPT) or bortezomib (VMP) have shown improved PFS and OS compared with MP alone [60, 61]. Recently, Rd has also been licensed for the treatment of non-ASCT eligible patients [62]. In the United States of America, also the monoclonal antibody daratumumab (anti-CD38) has been approved by the Food and Drug Administration for first line treatment of patients not eligible for ASCT, in combination with VMP.

Treatment for relapse/refractory patients include combinations of new-generation agents, such as carfilzomib [63], ixazomib [64] and elotuzumab [65], combined with Rd.

Moreover, patients previously treated with bortezomib and lenalidomide can benefit from pomalidomide or daratumumab alone or in combination with bortezomib and lenalidomide [66-68].

Pomalidomide is the third- generation IMiD, that can be used also in patients with renal failure. Carfilzomib, a second-generation PI used as single agent or in association with lenalidomide, is effective in relapsed myeloma, with a reduced neurotoxicity compared to bortezomib. However, it must be used carefully in patients with severe hypertension or cardiac disease. Ixazomib, another new PI, used in association with lenalidomide, has the advantage of oral administration, but can cause rash and diarrhea.

The monoclonal antibodody elotuzumab (anti-SLAMF7) plus Rd, has been recently approved for relapsed refractory MM. Daratumumab (anti-CD38) is licensed alone or in association with lenalidomide or bortezomib. Thanks to their good tolerability, these drugs can be especially indicated in the elderly. In particular, daratumumab seems to be the most effective drugs for heavily pre-treated patients, with surprising results as salvage treatment; however, patients with pulmonary disease must be strictly monitored for infusion reaction (bronchospasm, dyspnea, cough, dizziness etc.) that can appear during the administration.

In the relapse setting, for young, fit and high-risks patients, reduced-intensity allogeneic transplantation after ASCT can also be considered, if a suitable donor is available.

The choice of the best treatment for relapsed/refractory MM patients depends on:

- compliance, age, comorbidities,
- number and type of previous treatments, type of response, depth and length of response, side effects.
- aggressive disease, high-risks characteristics, plasma cells leukaemia or extramedullary involvement.

Response Evaluation

The response to treatment is evaluated according to the IMWG criteria. Response criteria are based on serum and urine assessment of monoclonal proteins and bone marrow assessment. However, given the high rates of CR seen in patients with new treatment approaches, new response categories have been recently defined for the identification of deeper and more sensitive responses. In the modern era of the MRD assessment by flow cytometry or gene sequencing and more sensitive imaging techniques the IMWG has defined new response categories of MRD negativity, with or without imaging-based absence of extramedullary disease [69].

Conclusion

Nowadays, the wide range of drugs available allows to choose between different combinations for the treatment of MM patients. However, the choice of the best schedule cannot be so obvious.

Numerous factors should be considered:

- patient's characteristics such as age, performance status, comorbidities, compliance and potential caregivers;
- disease characteristics such as high-risks factors, aggressive disease, plasma cells leukaemia or extramedullary involvement;
- (in case of relapse/refractory MM) the number and type of previous treatments, type of response, depth and length of response, side effects.

Unfortunately, there is not always a uniform and unanimous approach on the choice of the best treatment. Moreover, if we considered that a MM patient will face numerous relapses during the course of his disease and, as a consequence, numerous lines of therapy, it is very important to evaluate the type of treatment considering also the need of eventual further therapy in the future (for example, if we choose lenalidomide for the treatment of a patient we must considered that, if this patient will have a progression of disease during this course, we could not use drug combinations with lenalidomide for the next therapy).

There is not a uniform consensus also on when to start a new treatment (at biochemical relapse or clinical relapse).

Finally, as mentioned above, there are different opinions about the role of ASCT, especially in the era of the new drugs.

Therefore, it must be necessary to draw homogeneous therapeutic guidelines to identify the best sequence of treatment to adopt during the course of the disease and also the precise timing.

Maybe, a deeper characterization of patients (by phenotype, cytogenetic and molecular biology) and the evaluation of MRD would better stratify our patients and guide the physician in the choice of the best treatment, according to risk categories or to particular biological characteristics.

REFERENCES

[1] Kyle RA, Larson DR, Therneau TM, Dispenzieri A, Kumar S, Cerhan JR, et al. Long-term follow-up of monoclonal gammopathy of undetermined significance. *N Engl J Med.* 2018 Jan 18;378(3):241-249. doi: 10.1056/NEJMoa1709974.

[2] Lakshman A, Rajkumar SV, Buadi FK, Binder M, Gertz MA, Lacy MQ, et al. Risk stratification of smoldering multiple myeloma incorporating revised IMWG diagnostic criteria. *Blood Cancer J.* 2018 Jun 12;8(6):59. doi: 10.1038/s41408-018-0077-4.

[3] Mateos MV, Hernandex MH, Giraldo P, de la Rubia J, de Arriba F, Corral LL, et al. Lenalidomide plus dexamethasone versus observation in patients with high-risk smouldering multiple myeloma (QuiRedex): long-term follow-up a randomised, controlled, phase 3 trial. *Lancet Oncol.* 2016 Aug;17(8):1127-1136. doi: 10.1016/S1470-2045(16)30124-3.

[4] Ghobrial IM, Badros AZ, Vredenburgh JJ, Matous J, Caola AM, Savell A, et al. Phase II trial of combination of elotuzumab, lenalidomide, and dexamethasone in high-risk smoldering multiple myeloma. *58th American Society of Hematology* (ASH) 2016, 2016 Dec 3-6, San Diego, CA, USABlood. 2016;128(22):976–976.

[5] Korde N, Roschewski M, Zingone A, Kwok M, Manasanch EE, Bhutani M, et al. Treatment with carfilzomib-lenalidomide-dexamethasone with lenalidomide extension in patients with smoldering or newly diagnosed multiple myeloma. *JAMA Oncol.* 2015 Sep;1(6):746-54. doi: 10.1001/jamaoncol.2015.2010.

[6] National Cancer Institute. *Surveillance epidemiology and end results program. SEER stat fact sheets on multiple myeloma.* (internet), Bethesda (MD), National Cancer Institute, 2016 [cited April 24, 2013]. Available from: https://seer.cancer.gov/statfacts/html/mulmy.html.

[7] Pilarski LM, Piotrowska-Krezolak M, Gibney DJ, Winger L, Winger C, Mant MJ, et al. Specificity repertoire of lymphocytes from multiple myeloma patients. I. High frequency of B cells specific for

idiotypic and F(ab')2-region determinants on immunoglobulin. *J ClinImmunol.* 1985 Jul;5(4):275-84.

[8] Berenson J, Wong R, Kim K, Brown N, Lichtenstein A. Evidence for peripheral blood B lymphocyte but not T lymphocyte involvement in multiple myeloma. *Blood.* 1987 Nov;70(5):1550-3.

[9] Corradini P, Voena C, Omedè P, Astolfi M, Boccadoro M, Dalla-Favera R, et al. Detection of circulating tumor cells in multiple myeloma by a PCR-based method. *Leukemia.* 1993 Nov;7(11):1879-82.

[10] Kawano M, Hirano T, Matsuda T, Taga T, Horii Y, Iwato K, et al. Autocrine generation and requirement of BSF/IL-6 for human multiple myeloma. *Nature.* 1988 Mar 3;332(6159):83-5.

[11] Klein B, Zhang XG, Jourdan M, Content J, Houssiau F, Aarden L, et al. Paracrine rather than autocrine regulation of myeloma-cell growth and differentiation by interleukin-6. *Blood.* 1989 Feb;73(2):517-26.

[12] Hata H, Xiao H, Petrucci MT, Woodliff J, Chang R, Epstein J. Interleukin-6 gene expression in multiple myeloma: a characteristic of immature tumor cells. *Blood.* 1993 Jun 15;81(12):3357-64.

[13] Hardin J, MacLeod S, Grigorieva I, Chang R, Barlogie B, Xiao H, et al. Interleukin-6 prevents dexamethasone-induced myeloma cell death. *Blood.* 1994 Nov 1;84(9):3063-70.

[14] Carter A, Merchav S, Silvian-Draxler I, Tatarsky I. The role of interleukin-1 and tumor necrosis factor- (alpha) in human multiple myeloma. *Br J Haematol.* 1990 Apr;74(4):424-31.

[15] Roodman GD. Pathogenesis of myeloma bone disease. *Leukemia.* 2009 Mar;23(3):435-41. doi: 10.1038/leu.2008.336.

[16] Hideshima T, Mitsiades C, Tonon G, Richardson PG, Anderson KC. Under- standing multiple myeloma pathogenesis in the bone marrow to identify new therapeutic targets. *Nat Rev Cancer.* 2007 Aug; 7(8):585-98.

[17] Kuehl WM, Bergsagel PL. Multiple myeloma: evolving genetic events and host interactions. *Nat Rev Cancer.* 2002 Mar;2(3):175-87.

[18] Bergsagel PL, Kuehl WM. Molecular pathogenesis and a consequent classification of multiple myeloma. *J Clin Oncol.* 2005 Sep 10;23(26):6333-8.

[19] Avet-Loiseau, H., Attal, M., Moreau, P., Charbonnel, C., Garban, F., Hulin, C., et al. Genetic abnormalities and survival in multiple myeloma: the experience of the Intergroupe Francophone du Myélome. *Blood.* 2007 Apr 15;109(8):3489-95.

[20] Sonneveld, P., Avet-Loiseau, H., Lonial, S., Usmani, S., Siegel, D., Anderson KC, et al. Treatment of multiple myeloma with high-risk cytogenetics: a consensus of the International Myeloma Working Group.*Blood.* 2016 Jun 16;127(24):2955-62. doi: 10.1182/blood-2016-01-631200.

[21] Durie B. G., Salmon S. E. A clinical staging system for multiple myeloma correlation of measured myeloma cell mass with presenting clinical features, response to treatment, and survival. *Cancer.* 1975 Sep;36(3):842-54.

[22] Greipp, P. R., Katzmann, J. A, O'Fallon, W. M., Kyle, R. A. Value of beta 2-microglobulin level and plasma cell labeling indices as prognostic factors in patients with newly diagnosed myeloma. *Blood.* 1988 Jul;72(1):219-23.

[23] Battaille, R., Boccadoro, M., Klein, B., Durie, B., Pileri, A. C-Reactice Protein and β-2 microglobulin produce a simple and powerful myeloma staging system. *Blood.* 1992 Aug 1;80(3):733-7.

[24] Greipp, P. R., San Miguel, J., Durie, B. G., Crowley, J. J., Barlogie, B., Bladé, J., et al. International staging system for multiple myeloma. *J Clin Oncol.* 2005 May 20;23(15):3412-20.

[25] Palumbo, A., Avet-Loiseau, H., Oliva, S., Lokhorst, H. M, Goldschmidt H, Rosinol L, et al. Revised International Staging System for multiple myeloma: a report from International Myeloma Working Group. *J Clin Oncol.* 2015 Sep 10;33(26):2863-9. doi: 10.1200/JCO.2015.61.2267.

[26] Dispenzieri, A., Kyle, R., Merlini, G., Miguel, J. S., Ludwig, H., Hajek, R., et al. International MyelomaWorking Group guidelines for serum-free light chain analysis in multiple myeloma and related

disorders. *Leukemia.* 2009 Feb;23(2):215-24. doi: 10.1038/leu. 2008.307.

[27] Avet-Loiseau H. Role of genetics in prognostication in myeloma. *Best Pract Res Clin Haematol.* 2007 Dec;20(4):625-35.

[28] Terpos E., Moulopoulos L. A., Dimopoulos, M. A. Advances in imaging and the management of myeloma bone disease. *J Clin Oncol.* 2011 May 10;29(14):1907-15. doi: 10.1200/JCO.2010. 32.5449.

[29] Zamagni, E., Nanni, C., Patriarca, F., Englaro, E., Castellucci, P., Geatti, O., et al. A prospective comparison of 18F- fluoro-deoxyglucose positron emission tomography-computed tomography, magnetic resonance imaging and whole-body planar radiographs in the assessment of bone disease in newly diagnosed multiple myeloma. *Haematologica.* 2007;92(1):50-55.

[30] Zamagni E, Patriarca F, Nanni C, Zannetti B, Englaro E, Pezzi A, et al. Prognostic relevance of 18-F FDG PET/CT in newly diagnosed multiple myeloma patients treated with up-front autologous transplantation. *Blood.* 2011 Dec 1;118(23):5989-95. doi: 10.11 82/blood-2011-06-361386.

[31] Rajkumar S. V., Dimopoulos, M. A., Palumbo, A., Blade, J., Merlini, G., Mateos, M. V., et al. International Myeloma Working Group updated criteria for the diagnosis of multiple myeloma. *Lancet Oncol.* 2014 Nov;15(12):e538-48. doi: 10.1016/S1470-2045(14)70442-5.

[32] Attal, M., Harousseau, J. L., Stoppa, A. M., Sotto, J. J., Fuzibet, J. G., Rossi, J. F., et al. A prospective, randomized trial of autologous bone marrow transplantation and chemotherapy in multiple myeloma. Intergroupe Francais du Myelome. *N Engl J Med.* 1996;335(2):91-97.

[33] Child, J. A., Morgan, G. J., Davies, F. E., Owen, R. G., Bell, S. E., Hawkins K., et al. High-dose chemotherapy with hematopoietic stem-cellrescue for multiple myeloma. *N Engl J Med.* 2003;348(19):1875-1883.

[34] Harousseau J. L., Mathiot C., Attal M., Marit G., Caillot D., Hullin, C., et al. Bortezomib/dexamethasone versus VAD as induction prior to autologous stem cell transplantion (ASCT) in previously untreated multiple myeloma (MM): Updated data from IFM 2005/01 trial. 44th Annual Meeting of the American Society of Clinical Oncology (ASCO) 2008, 2008 May 30 - June 03, Chicago, Illinois;USA. *J Clin Oncol.* 2008;26(15):8505.

[35] Harousseau, J. L., Attal, M., Avet-Loiseau, H., Marit, G., Caillot, D., Mohty, M., et al. Bortezomib plus dexamethasone is superior to vincristine plus doxorubicin plus dexamethasone as induction treatment prior to autologous stem-cell transplantation in newly diagnosed multiple myeloma: results of the IFM 2005-01 phase III trial. *J Clin Oncol.* 2010 Oct 20;28(30):4621-9. doi: 10.1200/JCO. 2009.27.9158.

[36] Sonneveld P, Schmidt-Wolf IG, van der Holt B, El Jarari L, Bertsch U, Salwender H, et al. Bortezomib induction and maintenance treatment in patients with newly diagnosed multiple myeloma: results of the randomized phase III HOVON-65/ GMMG-HD4 trial. *J Clin Oncol.* 2012 Aug 20;30(24):2946-55. doi: 10.1200/JCO.20 11.39.6820.

[37] Cavo M, Zamagni E, Tosi P, Tacchetti P, Cellini C, Cangini D, et al. Superiority of thalidomide and dexamethasone over vincristine doxorubicin dexamethasone (VAD) as primary therapy in preparation for autologous transplantation for multiple myeloma. *Blood.* 2005 Jul 1;106(1):35-9.

[38] Macro M, Divine M, Uzunhan Y, Jaccard A, Bouscary D, Leblond V, et al. Dexamethasone thalidomide (Dex/Thal) compared to VAD as a pre-transplant treatment in newly diagnosed multiple myeloma (MM): a randomized trial. *48th Annual Meeting of the American Society of Hematology* (ASH) 2006, 2006 Dec 9-12, Orlando, FL; USA. Blood. 2006;108(11):57.

[39] Cavo M, Di Raimondo F, Zamagni E, Patriarca F, Tacchetti P, Casulli AF, et al. Short term thalidomide incorporated into double autologous stem-cell transplantation improbe outcomes compared

with double autotransplantation for multiple myeloma. *J ClinOncol.* 2009 Oct 20;27(30):5001-7. doi: 10.1200/JCO.2009.22.7389.

[40] Rajkumar SV, Jacobus S, Callander N, Fonseca R, Vesole D, Williams MV, et al. Randomized trial of lenalidomide plus high-dose dexamethasone versus lenalidomide plus low-dose dexamethasone in newly diagnosed myeloma (E4A03), a trial coordinated by the Eastern Cooperative Oncology Group: Analysis of response, survival, and outcome wi.*44th Annual Meeting of the American Society of Clinical Oncology* (ASCO) 2008, 2008 May 30 - June 03, Chicago, Illinois;USA. *J ClinOncol.* 2008;26(15):504.

[41] Cavo M, Tacchetti P, Patriarca F, Petrucci MT, Pantani L, Galli M, et al. Bortezomib, thalidomide and dexamethasone compared with thalidomide and dexamethasone as induction before and consolidation therapy after double autologous stem cell transplantation in newly diagnosed multiple myeloma: results from a randomized phase III study. *Lancet.* 2010 Dec 18;376(9758):2075-85. doi: 10.1016/S0140-6736(10)61424-9.

[42] Rosiñol L, Cibeira MT, Mateos MV, Martinez J, Oriol A, Teruel AI, et al. A phase III PETHEMA/GEM study of induction therapy prior autologous stem cell transplantation in multiple myeloma: superiority of VTD (bortezomib/thalidomide/dexamethasone) over TD and VBMCP/VBAD plus bortezomib. *52nd Annual Meeting of the American Society of Hematology* (ASH) 2010, 2010 Dec 4-7, Orlando, FL; USA. Blood 2010,116(21):307.

[43] Rosiñol L, Oriol A, Teruel AI, Hernández D, López-Jiménez J, de la Rubia J, et al. Superiority of bortezomib, thalidomide, and dexamethasone (VTD) as induction pretransplantation therapy in multiple myeloma: a randomized phase 3 PETHEMA/GEM study. *Blood.* 2012 Aug 23;120(8):1589-96.

[44] Kumar SK, Rajkumar SV, Dispenzieri A, Lacy MQ, Hayman SR, Buadi FK, et al. Improved survival in multiple myeloma and the impact of novel therapies. *Blood.* 2008 Mar 1;111(5):2516-20.

[45] National Cancer Comprehensive Network. *NCCN Clinical practice guidelines in oncology: multiplemyeloma.* http://wwwnccnorg/professionals/physician_gls/PDF/myelomapdf.

[46] Cavo M, Rajkumar SV, Palumbo A, Moreau P, Orlowski R, Bladé J, et al. International Myeloma Working Group consensus approach to the treatment of multiple myeloma patients who are candidates for autologous stem cell transplantation. *Blood.* 2011 Jun 9;117(23):6063-73. doi: 10.1182/blood-2011-02-297325.

[47] Moreau P, Avet-Loiseau H, Harousseau JL, Attal M. Current trends in autologous stem-cell transplantation for myeloma in the era of novel therapies. *J Clin Oncol.* 2011 May 10;29(14):1898-906. doi: 10.1200/JCO.2010.32.5878.

[48] Kumar S, Flinn I, Richardson PG, Hari P, Callander N, Noga SJ, et al. Randomized, multicenter, phase 2 study (EVOLUTION) of combinations of bortezomib, dexamethasone, cyclophosphamide, and lenalidomide in previously untreated multiple myeloma. *Blood.* 2012 May 10;119(19):4375-82. doi: 10.1182/blood-2011-11-395749.

[49] Ludwig H, Viterbo L, Greil R, Masszi T, Spicka I, Shpilberg O, et al. Randomized phase II study of bortezomib, thalidomide, and dexamethasone with or without cyclophosphamide as induction therapy in previously untreated multiple myeloma. *J Clin Oncol.* 2013 Jan 10;31(2):247-55. doi: 10.1200/JCO.2011.39.5137.

[50] Kumar SK, Lacy MQ, Dispenzieri A, Buadi FK, Hayman SR, Dingli D, et al. Early versus delayed autologous transplantation after immunomodulatory agents-based induction therapy in patients with newly diagnosed multiple myeloma. *Cancer.* 2012 Mar 15;118(6):1585-92. doi: 10.1002/cncr.26422.

[51] Dunavin NC1, Wei L, Elder P, Phillips GS, Benson DM Jr, Hofmeister CC, et al. Early versus delayed autologous stem cell transplant in patients receiving novel therapies for multiple myeloma. *Leuk Lymphoma.* 2013 Aug;54(8):1658-64. doi: 10.3109/10428194.2012.751528.

[52] Attal M, Lauwers-Cances V, Hulin C, Facon T, Caillot D, Escoffre M, et al. Autologous transplantation for multiple myeloma in the era

of new drugs: a phase III study of the Intergroupe Francophone du Myelome (IFM/DFCI 2009 Trial).*57th Annual Meeting of the American Society of Hematology* (ASH), 2015 Dec 5-8, Orlando, CA; USA. Blood. 2015;126(23):391.

[53] Gay F, Magarotto V, Petrucci MT, Di Raimondo F, Pour L, Caravita T, et al. Autologous transplantation versus cyclophosphamide-lenalidomide-prednisone followed by lenalidomide-prednisone versus lenalidomide maintenance in multiple myeloma: long-term results of a phase III trial. *57th Annual Meeting of the American Society of Hematology* (ASH) 2015, 2015 Dec5-8, Orlando, CA; USA. Blood. 2015;126(23):392.

[54] Palumbo A, Cavallo F, Gay F, Di Raimondo F, Ben Yehuda D, Petrucci MT, et al. Autologous transplantation and maintenance therapy in multiple myeloma. *N Engl J Med.* 2014 Sep 4;371(10):895-905. doi: 10.1056/NEJMoa1402888.

[55] Attal M, Harousseau JL, Facon T, Guilhot F, Doyen C, Fuzibet JG,et al. Single versus double autologous stem-cell transplantation for multiple myeloma. *N Engl J Med.* 2003 Dec 25;349(26):2495-502.

[56] Cavo M, Tosi P, Zamagni E, Cellini C, Tacchetti P, Patriarca F, et al. Prospective, randomized study of single compared with double autologous stem cell transplantation for multiple myeloma: bologna 96 clinical study. *J Clin Oncol.* 2007 Jun 10;25(17):2434-41.

[57] Harousseau JL. Hematopoietic stem cell transplantation in multiple myeloma. *J Natl Compr Canc Netw.* 2009 Oct;7(9):961-70.

[58] Cavo M, Salwender H, Rosiñol L, Moreau P, Petrucci MT, Blau IW, et al. Double vs single autologous stem cell transplantation after bortezomib-based induction regimens for multiple myeloma: an integrated analysis of patient-level data from Phase European III Studies Clinically Relevant. *55th Annual Meeting of the American Society of Hematology* (ASH) 2013, 2013 Dec 7-10,New Orleans, Louisiana; USA. Blood. 2013;122(21):767.

[59] Martino M, Recchia AG, Fedele R, Neri S, Vincelli ID, Moscato T, et al. The role of tandem stem cell transplantation for multiple

myeloma patients. *Expert Opin Biol Ther.* 2016;16(4):515-34. doi: 10.1517/14712598.2016.1136285.

[60] Fayers PM, Palumbo A, Hulin C, Waage A, Wijermans P, Beksaç M, et al. Thalidomide for previously untreated elderly patients with multiple myeloma: meta-analysis of 1685 individual patient data from 6 randomized clinical trials. *Blood.* 2011 Aug 4;118(5):1239-47. doi: 10.1182/blood-2011-03-341669.

[61] San Miguel JF, Schlag R, Khuageva NK, Dimopoulos MA, Shpilberg O, Kropff M, et al. Bortezomib plus melphalan and prednisone for initial treatment of multiple myeloma. *N Engl J Med.* 2008 Aug 28;359(9):906-17. doi: 10.1056/NEJMoa0801479.

[62] Facon T, Dimopoulos MA, Dispenzieri A, Catalano JV, Belch A, Cavo M, et al. Final analysis of overall survival from the First trial. *58th American Society of Hematology* (ASH) 2016, 2016 Dec 3-6, San Diego, CA, USA. *Blood.* 2016;128(22):653.

[63] Stewart, K. A., Rajkumar, S. V., Dimopoulos, M. A., Masszi, T., Špička, I., Oriol, A., et al. Carfilzomib, lenalidomide, and dexamethasone for relapsed multiple myeloma. *N Engl J Med.* 2015 Jan 8;372(2):142-52. doi: 10.1056/NEJMoa1411321

[64] Moreau, P., Masszi, T., Grzasko, N., Bahlis, N. J, Hansson, M., Pour, L., et al. Oral ixazomib, lenalidomide, and dexamethasone for multiple myeloma. *N Engl J Med.* 2016 Apr 28;374(17):1621-34. doi: 10.1056/NEJMoa1516282.

[65] Lonial, S., Dimopoulos, M., Palumbo, A., White, D., Grosicki, S., Spicka, I., et al. Elotuzumab therapy for relapsed or refractory multiple myeloma. *N Engl J Med.* 2015 Aug 13;373(7):621-31. doi: 10.1056/NEJMoa1505654.

[66] Lonial, S., Weiss, B. M., Usmani, S. Z., Singhal, S., Chari, A., Bahlis, N. J., et al. Daratumumab monotherapy in patients with treatment-refractory multiple myeloma (SIRIUS): an open-label, randomised, phase 2 trial. *Lancet.* 2016 Apr 9;387(10027):1551-60. doi: 10.1016/S0140-6736(15)01120-4.

[67] Spencer, A., Lentzsch, S., Weisel, K., Avet-Loiseau, H., Mark, T. M., Spicka, I., et al. Daratumumab plus bortezomib and

dexamethasone versus bortezomib and dexamethasone in relapsed or refractory multiple myeloma: updated analysis of CASTOR. *Haematologica.* 2018 Sep 20. pii: haematol.2018.194118. doi: 10.3324/haematol.20 18.194118.

[68] Dimopoulos, M. A., San-Miguel, J., Belch, A., White, D., Benboubker, L., Cook, G., et al. Daratumumab plus lenalidomide and dexamethasone versus lenalidomide and dexamethasone in relapsed or refractory multiple myeloma: updated analysis of POLLUX. *Haematologica.* 2018 Sep 20. pii: haematol.2018.194282. doi: 10.3324/haematol. 2018.194282.

[69] Kumar, S., Paiva, B., Anderson, K. A.., Durie, B4, Landgren, O5, Moreau, P., et al. International Myeloma Working Group consensus criteria for response and minimal residual disease assessment in multiple myeloma. *Lancet Oncol.* 2016 Aug;17(8):e328-e346. doi: 10.101 6/S1470-2045(16)30206-6.

In: Advances in Health and Disease
Editor: Lowell T. Duncan
ISBN: 978-1-53616-380-3

Chapter 3

HYPERBARIC OXYGEN THERAPY IN SUDDEN SENSORINEURAL HEARING LOSS

Sema Zer Toros[1], MD, Omer Cagatay Ertugay[2], MD and Cigdem Kalaycik Ertugay[3,*], MD

[1]Professor, Haydarpasa Numune Education and Research Hospital, Department of Otorhinolaryngology/Head and Neck Surgery, Istanbul, Turkey

[2]Specialist, Haydarpasa Numune Education and Research Hospital, Department of Otorhinolaryngology/Head and Neck Surgery, Istanbul, Turkey

[3]Associate Professor, Istanbul Education and Research Hospital, Department of Otorhinolaryngology/Head and Neck Surgery, Istanbul, Turkey

ABSTRACT

Sudden sensorineural hearing loss (SSNHL) is a common clinical entity and defined as a rapid onset of hearing impairment, occurring

---

* Corresponding Author's Email: ckalaycik@gmail.com.

within three days. It has an audiometric criteria identified as a decrease in hearing of at least 30 dB over three contiguous test frequencies in one or both ears. It has a significant effect on quality of life. As the 88% of SSNHL cases is idiopathic at presentation, there is usually no known exact specific etiologic factor. However, multiple reasons such as vascular compromise and associated cochlear ischemia or viral etiologies, etc. have been presumed and the treatment modalities have been empiric. Although oral steroid therapy is the mainstay treatment in clinical practice, in most of the centers, several different treatment modalities proposed in the literature. Hyperbaric oxygen therapy (HBOT), which has been used for SSNHL treatment since 1979, exposes a patient to 100% oxygen at a pressure level higher than 1 atmosphere absolute in a specially designed sealed chamber. This facilitates a delivery of increased partial pressure of oxygen to the tissues. Based on this fact, it is thought that HBOT may prevent damage caused from ischemia by improving the supply of oxygen to the inner ear and result in an improvement in hearing. This review focuses on the benefits and harms of HBOT in treating SSNHL.

Keywords: Sudden sensorineural hearing loss, hyperbaric oxygen therapy, hearing impairment

INTRODUCTION

Sudden sensorineural hearing loss (SSNHL) is a common clinical entity and defined as a rapid onset of hearing impairment in one or both ears, occurring within three days. It has an audiometric criteria identified as a decrease in hearing of at least 30 dB over three contiguous test frequencies in one or both ears. Patients usually admit to the emergency department because of the frightening symptoms such as aural fullness, tinnitus or vertigo. It affects 4000 new people per year in the United States [1-2]. Approximately 88% of SSNHL cases is idiopathic at presentation. However, multiple reasons such as vascular compromise and associated cochlear ischemia, viral etiologies, autoimmune, trauma, schwannoma, demyelinating disease, etc. have been presumed [3]. If the clinicians cannot identify the reason, it is named as idiopathic SSNHL and the treatment is empiric. The exact spontaneous recovery rate cannot be determined, because most of the patients seek medical care in the early period and are treated empirically. The reported rate of spontaneous recovery ranges from 32% to 65% [2, 4]. Although hearing aids are recommended in nonhealing patients with moderate or severe hearing loss, SSNHL has a significant effect on quality of life. There are various different treatment modalities such as systemic and intratympanic steroids, vasodilators, antiviral agents, diuretics, hyperbaric oxygen therapy (HBOT), etc. However, the exact efficacy of these treatments is not known due to the fact that clinicians cannot determine a definitive etiology in most of the cases. Although oral steroid therapy is the mainstay treatment in clinical practice in most of the centers, there are several randomized controlled studies for only HBOT [5-7].

INDICATIONS

The blood supply of inner ear and vestibulocochlear nerve is maintained by labyrinthine artery and also by diffusion through perilymph and cortilymph. The labyrinthine artery has no anastomosis. Therefore, cochlea is very sensitive to ischemia and cochlear hypoxia results in progressive degenerative changes, loss of neurons, and hearing loss.

Vascular compromise and associated cochlear ischemia is one of the possible etiologic factors of SSNHL. HBOT exposes a patient to 100% oxygen at a pressure level higher than 1 atmosphere absolute in a specially designed sealed chamber. This facilitates a delivery of increased partial pressure of oxygen to the tissues. Moreover, it may improve the host reaction against infection and ischemia by reducing hypoxia and edema due to its complex effects on immunity, oxygen transport, and hemodynamics [8]. Based on these facts, it is thought that HBOT may prevent damage caused from ischemia by improving the supply of oxygen to the inner ear, increasing the oxygen tension in perilymph and result in an improvement in hearing. The patency of labyrinthine artery and the rising rate of oxygen tension in perilymph influence the efficacy of HBOT in SSNHL [9].

The clinical guideline of The American Academy of Otolaryngology indicated that corticosteroids and HBOT are treatment options whereas other pharmacologic therapies such as antivirals, thrombolytics, vasodilators, vasoactive substances, or antioxidants should not be prescribed routinely by clinicians. The guideline stated that patient needs multiple 1- to 2-hour sessions (mostly 5 to 10 times) over days to weeks for HBOT which is expensive and the reports about HBOT had small number of patients and methodological shortcomings. However, they indicated that HBOT may have benefits according to the reported studies and offered HBOT as an adjunctive therapy. They emphasized that it may have better effect in the early period (within 3 months of the onset of SSNHL), younger patients (younger than 50-60 years), and patients with moderate to severe or severe to profound hearing loss [10].

SIDE EFFECTS AND COMPLICATIONS

The possible side effects of HBOT include oxygen poisoning, claustrophobia, temporary worsening of short-sightedness, and damage to sinuses, lungs, and ears due to the pressure changes [10]. The cochrane database review including seven randomized controlled trials, which evaluated the efficacy of HBOT on treatment of SSNHL, reported no systemic side effects [11]. The most common complication of HBOT is middle ear barotrauma [9]. Plafki et al. evaluated the complications and side effects of HBOT in 782 patients with 11,376 sessions. The indication of HBOT in this patients was various. They identified that ear pain or discomfort was the predominant complaint of patients which was seen in 17% of patients. They indicated that this is due to the difficultly equalizing pressure in the middle ear [12]. Fernau et al. evaluated the effect of HBOT on eustachian tube function in patients who undergone HBOT for several different indications and detected eustachian tube dysfunction in 45% of patients [13]. On the other hand, the complication rate in the patients undergoing HBOT for SSNHL is fewer. The concurrent use of systemic steroids might be the reason of this, because steroids may decrease the edema or inflammation which enhances the pressure equalization [10]. Pilgramm et al. reported that three of their participants who were performed HBOT for SSNHL were withdrawn the therapy due to the middle ear barotrauma [14]. Another study observed 6.25% ear or sinus barotrauma in 80 patients undergoing HBOT for SSNHL [15].

CONTRAINDICATIONS

The major contraindications include pneumothorax, severe reactive airways disease, severe congestive heart failure, concomitant doxorubicin or bleomycin therapy, and confinement anxiety [9].

RELATED ARTICLES

The first usage of HBOT in SSHNL in the literature was in 1979 [16]. Since that time, various studies have been performed [5-7, 11]. The improvement of hearing loss with HBOT was indicated in a cochrane database review but the certain level or clinical relevance of this improvement was not clear. This report reviewed seven trials published between 1985 and 2004 including 392 participants in whom 207 received HBOT and 185 was control. The dose of oxygen per treatment session varied between 1.5 and 2.5 ATA as a maximum oxygen pressure and the total course of treatment varied between 10 to 25 sessions in these randomized controlled studies included in this review. They determined the chance of a 25% increase following HBOT. They indicated that better results may be seen if the patient was treated within 2 weeks of acute onset and the amelioration may be associated with onset severity of the hearing loss [11].

Naiboglu et al. evaluated the effects of three treatment modalities which were intratympanic steroid, systemic steroid, and HBOT on SSNHL treatment. They indicated that patients with profound hearing loss might have better success rate if these three treatment modalities are applied together [17].

Ajduk et al. investigated 93 patients with SSNHL who did not get benefit from steroid therapy. Forty-three of these patients had undergone HBOT as a salvage therapy. They found that although patients with moderate hearing loss (≤60 dB) had improvement only at low frequencies (0.25 and 0.5 kHz), patients with severe hearing loss (>61 dB) had improvement at all frequencies [18].

Alimoglu et al. investigated the impact of HBOT as a salvage treatment of SSNHL by retrospectively reviewing the medical records of their patients who had received a 14-day course of failed oral corticosteroid therapy. They found that the mean gain of pure tone average was more prominent in lower frequencies (0.25 kHz and 0.5 kHz) than higher ones. They proposed that the reason might be the increased vulnerability of the basal turn of the cochlea to damage which leads to a lower predisposition to the recovery [19]. Similar to the report of Alimoglu et al., Muzzi et al. observed higher gains in lower frequencies in 19 patients who received 30 sessions of HBOT after failed medical treatment. However, they did not state the details of applied medical treatment [20].

On the other hand, Cekin et al. studied the efficacy of HBOT on SSNHL as an adjunctive treatment by treating 36 patients with HBOT with concomitant medical therapy with prednisolone (study group) and treating 21 patients with only prednisolone (control group). They compared these two patient groups. Although they found higher success rate in the study group, this difference was not statistically significant. They suggested HBOT as an alternative therapy only if the patients have contraindications for medical therapy such as peptic ulceration, hypertension, old age, etc. [21].

REFERENCES

[1] Byl F. M. Seventy-six cases of presumed sudden hearing loss occurring in 1973: prognosis and incidence. *Laryngoscope*. 1977;87(5, pt 1):817-825.

[2] Mattox D. E., Simmons F. B. Natural history of sudden sensorineural hearing loss. *Ann. Otol. Rhinol. Laryngol.* 1977;86(4, pt 1):463-480.

[3] Rauch S. D. Clinical practice: idiopathic sudden sensorineural hearing loss. *N. Engl. J. Med.* 2008;359(8):833-840.

[4] Conlin A. E., Parnes L. S. Treatment of sudden sensorineural hearing loss, II: a meta-analysis. *Arch. Otolaryngol. Head Neck Surg.* 2007;133(6):582-586.

[5] Narozny W., Kuczkowski J., Mikaszewski B. HBO effectively supports SSNHL therapy. *Eur. Arch. Otorhinolaryngol.* 2005; 262(2):163-4.

[6] Racic G., Maslovara S., Roje Z., et al. Hyperbaric oxygen in the treatment of sudden hearing loss. *ORL J. Otorhinolaryngol. Relat. Spec.* 2003;65(6):317-20.

[7] Horn C. E., Himel H. N., Selesnick S. H. Hyperbaric oxygen therapy for sudden sensorineural hearing loss: a prospective trial of patients failing steroid and antiviral treatment. *Otol. Neurotol.* 2005; 26(5):882-9.

[8] Gill A. L., Bell C. N. Hyperbaric oxygen: its uses, mechanisms of action and outcomes. *QJM*. 2004;97(7):385-395.

[9] Murphy-Lavoie H. M., Mutluoglu M. Hyperbaric, Sensorineural Hearing Loss. In: *StatPearls* [Internet]. Treasure Island (FL): StatPearls Publishing; 2019-2018 Oct 27.

[10] Stachler R. J., Chandrasekhar S. S., Archer S. M., et al. Clinical practice guideline: sudden hearing loss. *Otolaryngol. Head Neck Surg.* 2012; 146(3 Suppl.):S1-35.

[11] Bennett M. H., Kertesz T., Yeung P. Hyperbaric oxygen for idiopathic sudden sensorineural hearing loss and tinnitus. *Cochrane Database Syst. Rev.* 2007;1:CD004739.

[12] Plafki C., Peters P., Almeling M., Welslau W., Busch R. Complications and side effects of hyperbaric oxygen therapy. *Aviat. Space Environ. Med.* 2000;71(2):119-124.

[13] Fernau J. L., Hirsch B. E., Derkay C., Ramasastry S., Schaefer S. E. Hyperbaric oxygen therapy: effect on middle ear and eusta- chian tube function. *Laryngoscope*. 1992;102(1):48-52.

[14] Pilgramm M., Lamm H., Schumann K. Hyperbaric oxygen therapy in sudden deafness [Zur hyperbaren Sauerstofftherapie beim Hörsturz]. *Laryngologie, Rhinologie, Otologie* 1985;64(7):351-4.

[15] Korpinar S., Alkan Z., Yigit O., et al. Factors influencing the outcome of idiopathic sudden sensorineural hearing loss treated with hyperbaric oxygen therapy. *Eur. Arch. Otorhinolaryngol.* 2011;268(1):41-47.

[16] Goto F., Fujita T., Kitani Y., et al. Hyperbaric oxygen and stellate ganglion blocks for idiopathic sudden hearing loss. *Acta Otolaryngol.* 1979;88(5-6):335-42.

[17] Naiboğllu B., Külekçi S., Sürmeli M., Verim A., Kalaycik Ertugay Ç., İhvan Ö., Şeneldir L., Zer Toros S. Efficacy of multimodality approach to sudden hearing loss. *The Turkish Journal of Ear Nose and Throat*, 2015;25(2), 77-81.

[18] Ajduk J., Ries M., Trotic R., Marinac I., Vlatka K., Bedekovic V. Hyperbaric Oxygen Therapy as Salvage Therapy for Sudden Sensorineural Hearing Loss. *J. Int. Adv. Otol.* 2017;13(1):61-64.

[19] Alimoglu Y., Inci E. Is hyperbaric oxygen therapy a salvage treatment option for sudden sensorineural hearing loss? *J. Laryngol. Otol.* 2016 Oct;130(10):943-947.

[20] Muzzi E., Zennaro B., Visentin R., Soldano F., Sacilotto C. Hyperbaric oxygen therapy as salvage treatment for sudden sensorineural hearing loss: review of rationale and preliminary report. *J. Laryngol. Otol.* 2010;124:e2.

[21] Cekin E., Cincik H., Ulubil S. A., Gungor A. Effectiveness of hyperbaric oxygen therapy in management of sudden hearing loss. *J. Laryngol. Otol.* 2009;123(6):609-612.

In: Advances in Health and Disease
Editor: Lowell T. Duncan
ISBN: 978-1-53616-380-3

Chapter 4

SECONDARY, OFF-LABEL USES OF RUXOLITINIB

Julia Song[1,*], MD, Alice Song[2,†], MD, Trisa Palmares[1,‡], MD, Michael Song[2,§] and Harold Song[2,¶], MD

[1]Southern California Eye Physicians and Surgeons, Pasadena, CA, US

[2]Center for Oculofacial and Orbital Surgery, Los Alamitos, CA, US

ABSTRACT

Introduction: Since its advent, ruxolitinib has been shown to be a very effective treatment for myelofibrosis and polycythemia vera. Drugs can sometimes have uses beyond the official approved indication.

* Corresponding Author's Email: jsongmd@drsongvision.com.
† Email: asongmd@drsongvision.com.
‡ Email: trisa@drsongvision.com.
§ Email: Mike@drsongvision.com.
¶ Email: juliasongmd@gmail.com.

Hypereosinophilic syndrome (HES) is a hematologic disorder in which the eosinophils overproliferate. JAK inhibitors have also demonstrated efficacy in treating HES, as well as in the treatments of alopecia and madarosis.

Method: Review of literature

Conclusion: Ruxolitinib has beneficial effects in treating other conditions, considered off-label. These include HES, alopecia areata, and madarosis. Physicians and patients should be aware of the side effects of these JAK inhibitors. Further investigation is needed to ascertain whether ruxolitinib or other interleukin inhibitors can aid in the treatment of additional conditions.

Keywords: hypereosinophilic syndrome, ruxolitinib, alopecia, madarosis, JAK, Janus Kinase

Introduction

Ruxolitinib is a Janus kinase (JAK) inhibitor approved for the treatment of myelofibrosis and polycythemia vera. It has been proven to be effective in other indications, used off-label. These include hypereosinophilic syndrome (HES), alopecia areata, madarosis, vitiligo, and eczema.

Discussion

Ruxolitinib is an effective immunotherapy for the treatment of bone marrow conditions. It has also been proven to be efficacious in other conditions, for which it is not approved. These are known as off-label indications. These include hypereosinophilic syndrome, alopecia areata, and madarosis. The medication is fairly well-tolerated. Physicians and patients should be aware of the potential side effects of these JAK inhibitors. Further investigation is needed to ascertain whether ruxolitinib or other interleukin inhibitors can aid in the treatment of other conditions.

Hypereosinophilic syndrome (HES) is a rare hematologic disorder in which the eosinophils proliferate. The eosinophils infiltrate and damage multiple organs. Without treatment, the condition is fatal, usually due to cardiac dysfunction, particularly left ventricular dysfunction. Causes of reactive eosinophilia include allergic and hypersensitivity reactions, drug allergies, cytokine therapy (recombinant human interleukin), cutaneous disorders, connective tissue diseases, collagen vascular disorders, parasitic infections, immunodeficiency disorders, sarcoidosis, and neoplasms, such as Hodgkin's and non-Hodgkin's lymphomas and acute lymphoplastic leukemia. Various hematopoietic neoplasms that demonstrate blood eosinophilis are B-cell and T-cell non-Hodgkin's lymphomas, chronic myeloproliferative disorders such as chronic myelogenous leukemia, chronic eosinophilic leukemia, and systemic mast cell disease. (Acute myeloproliferative disorders include acute myelomonocyticleukemia (AML) with eosinophilia, acute lymphoblastic leukemia with eosinophilia).

Ruxolitinib is a janus kinase (JAK) inhibitor. Ruxolitinib inhibits dysregulated JAK signaling associated with cancer. There exist JAK1, JAK2, and JAK3 inhibitors. JAK1 and JAK2 are responsible for signaling transducers and activators of transcription (STATs) to cytokine receptors, leading to modulation of gene expression.

In 2011, ruxolitinib was approved for myelofibrosis (MF) and reducing splenomegaly. In 2014, it was also approved for polycythemia vera. Patients with graft versus host disease also benefit from the medication. In 2012, another JAK inhibitor (JAK1 and JAK3), tofacitinib, was approved for rheumatoid arthritis. Tofacitinib was approved for psorasiatic arthritis in 2018. The mechanism involves downregulation of tumor necrosis factor (TNF) and interleukin-17 (IL-17).

Ruxolitinib (Jakafi®) is off-label for HES but has been reported to be extremely successful. It has been also reported to aid in dermatologic conditions, such as refractory alopecia areata, vitiligo, and eczema. It has also been reported to aid in eyelash growth.

HES is a potentially fatal hematologic condition that requires prompt diagnosis and treatment. If untreated, patients will succumb to death, usually due to left ventricular cardiac dysfunction. Patients are extremely uncomfortable due to continual pruritus. JAK2 mutations have been identified as a marker which can be targeted by specific drugs, particularly ruxolitinib [1, 2, 3, 4].

Ruxolitinib (Jakafi®) was approved by the U.S. Food and Drug Administration (FDA) on November 16, 2011, as the first and only treatment for intermediate- or high-risk myelofibrosis (MF) [5]. It has been shown to aid in MF, polycythemia vera, and essential thrombocytopenia, specifically splenomegaly reduction [6].

Ruxolitinib is classified as a biologic response modifier, a signal transduction inhibitor, and a kinase inhibitor. Ruxolitinib, like inhibitors in its class, acts intracellularly against a specific signaling pathway. In this case, ruxolitinib targets the JAK-STAT signaling pathway, inhibiting JAK1 and JAK2. It is the first drug approved by the FDA to target this pathway. By inhibiting the two JAK kinases, ruxolitinib interrupts the signal sent to HPCS (hematopoietic progenitor cell) that would have resulted in unnecessary hematopoiesis, thus preventing additional marrow fibrosis. The most common adverse reactions to ruxolitinib are hematologic, specifically thrombocytopenia and anemia, both of which are dose-related. Although neutropenia is less common, thrombocytopenia and anemia (all grades) occurred in 70% and 96% of patients taking ruxolitinib.

Alopecia areata is an autoimmune condition of the hair follicles. The body attacks its own anagen hair follicles. T cell lymphocytes cluster near the hair follicles, resulting in inflammation and hair loss. This results in bald patches, usually of the scalp and beard but may affect any part of the body. It affects 0.1%-0.2% of the population and is indiscriminant towards gender.

Madarosis is a term which was originally coined to denote loss of eyelashes due to destruction of hair follicles, but now encompasses the loss of cilia of both eyelashes and eyebrows [7]. It can occur following trauma, surgery, or chemotherapy. It can also be a result of a psychiatric condition, trichotillomania, in which patients have an irresistible urge to pull on their eyelashes.

Madarosis can be divided into 2 groups: Scarring or non-scarring depending upon the etiology. Appropriate diagnosis is essential for management. Follicular unit transplantation has been found to be a useful method of treating scarring madarosis.

Madarosis can be disfiguring and cause morbidity. Topical prostaglandins, which have been used in the treatment of glaucoma, have been utilized for eyelash growth for both cosmetic reasons and for medical conditions [8 - 19]. There was one case of prostaglandin-induced poliosis [12]. Topical prostaglandins may cause unwanted side effects, such as deepening of the superior sulcus and fat atrophy; there was found to be enhancement of the eyelid crease in Asian eyelids and decrease in proptosis [20 - 23].

Oral ruxolitinib and other JAK inhibitors, tofacitinib, have been shown to aid in the treatment of alopecia areata, alopecia universalis, and alopecia totalis [24 - 30] as well as psoriasis [31]. A 77 year-old male with HES taking ruxolitinib was found to have an increase in thickness of his eyelashes [32].

Due to the above mentioned systemic side effects of oral ruxolitinib, topical ruxolitinib was developed recently. Topical ruxolitinib 0.6% cream bid has been proven to improve eyebrow and scalp hair growth [33].

Vitiligo is a long-term skin condition characterized by patches of the skin because the melanocytes die or stop producing pigment. Topical ruxolitinib was found to be efficacious in improving the appearance of vitiligo [34].

CONCLUSION

Oral ruxolitinib has secondary, off-label effects that may be beneficial. It can aid in alopecia areata, madarosis, and vitiligo. Care should be taken with oral ruxolitinib, as the medication has side effects. A review of all patients with MF treated with ruxolitinib to assess their facial and body hair may be warranted. Topical ruxolitinib cream may be useful; an ophthalmic drop or ointment or sustain-release form of the medication may be beneficial, targeted therapy in the future.

References

[1] Lierman, E., Selleslag, D., Smits, S., Billiet, J., Vandenberghe, P. (2012). Ruxolitinib inhibits transforming JAK2 fusion proteins in vitro and induces complete cytogenetic remission in t(8;9)(p22; p24)/PCM1-JAK2-positive chronic eosinophilic leukemia. *Blood.* 120(7):1529-1531.

[2] Rumi, E., Milosevic, J. D., Selleslag, D., Casetti, I., Lierman, E., Pietra, D., Cavalloni, C., Bellini, M., Milanesi, C., Dambruoso, I., Astori, C., Kralovics, R., Vandenberghe, P., Cazzola, M. (2015). Efficacy of ruxolitinib in myeloid neoplasms with PCM1-JAK2 fusion gene. *Ann Hematol.* Nov; 94(11):1927-8.

[3] Verstovsek, S., Mesa, R. A., Gotlib, J., Levy, R. S., Gupta, V., DiPersio, J. F., Catalano, J. V., Deininger, M., Miller, C., Silver, R. T., Talpaz, M., Winton, E. F., Harvey, J. H. Jr, Arcasoy, M. O., Hexner, E., Lyons, R. M., Paquette, R., Raza, A., Vaddi, K., Erickson-Viitanen, S., Koumenis, I. L., Sun, W., Sandor, V., Kantarjian, H. M. (2012). A double-blind, placebo controlled trial of ruxolitinib for myelofibrosis. *New England Journal of Medicine*. 366, 799–807.

[4] Schwaab, J., Umbach, R., Metzgeroth, G., Naumann, N., Jawhar, M., Sotlar, K., Horny, H. P., Gaiser, T., Hofmann, W. K., Schnittger, S., Cross, N. C., Fabarius, A., Reiter, A. (2015). KIT D816V and JAK2 V617F mutations are seen recurrently in hypereosinophilia of unknown significance. *Am J Hematol.* 90774-7.

[5] Incyte Corporation. (2011a). FDA approves Incyte's Jakafi® (ruxolitinib) for patients with myelofibrosis. Retrieved from http://investor.incyte.com/phoenix.zhtml?c=69764&p=irol-news Article&ID=1631201&highlight.

[6] Verstovsek, S. (2013). Ruxolitinib: an oral Janus kinase 1 and Janus kinase 2 inhibitor in the management of myelofibrosis. *Postgrad Med.* Jan; 125: 128-35.
[7] Duke-Elder, S., MacFaul, P. (1974). The ocular adnexa, part I: diseases of the eyelashes. In: Duke-Elder S, editor. *System of Ophthalmology.* Vol. 13. St Louis: CV Mosby; 373–90.
[8] Ahluwalia, G. S. (2013). Safety and efficacy of bimatoprost solution 0.03% topical application in patients with chemotherapy-induced eyelash loss. *J Investig Dermatol Symp Proc.* Dec; 16: S73-6.
[9] Fagien, S., Walt, J. G., Carruthers, J., Cox, S. E., Wirta, D., Weng, E., Beddingfield, F. C. 3rd. (2013). Patient-reported outcomes of bimatoprost for eyelash growth: results from a randomized, double-masked, vehicle-controlled, parallel-group study. *Aesthet Surg J.* Aug 1;33:789-98.
[10] Wand, M. (1997). Latanoprost and hyperpigmentation of eyelashes. *Arch Ophthalmol.* Sep; 115(9):1206-8.
[11] Strober, B. E., Potash, S., Grossman, M. E. (2001). Eyelash hypertrichosis in a patient treated with topical latanoprost. *Cutis.* Feb; 67:109-10.
[12] Chen, C. S., Wells, J., Craig, J. E. (2004). Topical prostaglandin F(2alpha) analog induced poliosis. *Am J Ophthalmol.* May; 137:965-6.
[13] Yan, g H. K., Park, K. H., Kim, T. W., Kim, D. M. (2009). Deepening of eyelid superior sulcus during topical travoprost treatment. *Jpn J Ophthalmol.* 53: 176-9.
[14] Moroi, S. E. (2010). Eyelash preservation during chemotherapy and topical prostaglandin therapy. *Arch Intern Med.* Jul 26; 170: 1269-70.
[15] Bikowski, J., Lau, E. G., Jacob, S. E. (2010). Eyelash growth: a beneficial side effect of prostaglandin analogues. *Cutis.* 85:187-8.
[16] Yoelin, S., Walt, J. G., Earl, M. (2010). Safety, effectiveness, and subjective experience with topical bimatoprost 0.03% for eyelash growth. *Dermatol Surg.* 36: 638-49.

[17] Cohen, J. L. (2010). Enhancing the growth of natural eyelashes: the mechanism of bimatoprost-induced eyelash growth. *Dermatol Surg.* 36: 1361-71.

[18] Cohen, J. L. (2010). Commentary: From serendipity to pilot study and then pivotal trial: bimatoprost topical for eyelash growth. *Dermatol Surg.* 36: 650-1.

[19] Bimatoprost 0.03% solution (latisse) for eyelash enhancement. *Med Lett Drugs Ther.* 2009 Jun 1;51(1313):43-4.

[20] Song, J., Song, A. (2012). Topical prostaglandin aids in forming crease in patients with incomplete lid crease. Poster. Asian Pacific Academy of Ophthalmology. April.

[21] Song, J. (2013). A medical approach to forming a complete eyelid crease. *Glaucoma Today.* Mar/Apr: 57-8.

[22] Song, J., Song, A., Song, M., Palmares, T. (2013). Oculoplastic and Orbital Effects of Topical Prostaglandins: Eyelid Crease Formation and Proptosis Reduction. Poster. American Society of Ophthalmic Plastic & Reconstructive Surgery. November 14.

[23] Faghihi, G., Andalib, F., Asilian, A. (2009). The efficacy of latanoprost in the treatment of alopecia areata of eyelashes and eyebrows. *Eur J Dermatol.* Nov-Dec; 19: 586-7.

[24] Mackay-Wiggan, J., Jabbari, A., Nguyen, N., Cerise, J. E., Clark, C., Ulerio, G., Furniss, M., Vaughan, R., Christiano, A. M., Clynes, R. (2016). Oral ruxolitinib induces hair regrowth in patients with moderate-to-severe alopecia areata. *JCI Insight.* Sep 22;1(15):e89790.

[25] Harris, J. E., Rashighi, M., Nguyen, N., Jabbari, A., Ulerio, G., Clynes, R., Christiano, A. M., Mackay-Wiggan, J. (2016). Rapid skin repigmentation on oral ruxolitinib in a patient with coexistent vitiligo and alopecia areata (AA). *J Am Acad Dermatol.* Feb; 74(2):370-1.

[26] Pieri, L., Guglielmelli, P., Vannucch, A. M. (2015). Ruxolitinib-induced reversal of alopecia universalis in a patient with essential thrombocythemia. *Am J Hematol.* 90:82-3.

[27] Xing, L., Dai, Z., Jabbari, A., Cerise, J. E., Higgins, C. A., Gong, W., de Jong, A., Harel, S., DeStefano, G. M., Rothman, L., Singh, P.,

Petukhova, L., Mackay-Wiggan, J., Christiano, A. M., Clynes R. (2014). Alopecia areata is driven by cytotoxic T lymphocytes and is reversed by JAK inhibition. *Nat Med.* Sep; 20(9):1043-9.

[28] Liu, L. Y., Craiglow, B. G., Dai, F., King, B. A. (2016). Tofacitinib for the treatment of severe alopecia areata and variants: A study of 90 patients. *J Am Acad Dermatol.* Nov 2.

[29] Craiglow, B. G., Liu, L. Y., King, B. A. (2016). Tofacitinib for the treatment of alopecia areata and variants in adolescents. *J Am Acad Dermatol.*

[30] Kennedy Crispin, M., Ko, J. M., Craiglow, B. G., Li, S., Shankar, G., Urban, J. R., Chen, J. C., Cerise, J. E., Jabbari, A., Winge, M. C., Marinkovich, M. P., Christiano, A. M., Oro, A. E., King, B. A. (2016). Safety and efficacy of the JAK inhibitor tofacitinib citrate in patients with alopecia areata. *JCI Insight.* Sep 22;1(15).

[31] Damsky, W., King, B. A. (2017). JAK inhibitors in dermatology: The promise of a new drug class. *J Am Acad Dermatol.* Apr; 76(4):736-744.

[32] Song J, Song A, Palmares T, Song M, Song H. (2017). Ruxolitinib found to cause eyelash growth: a case report. *J Med Case Rep.* 2017 Jul 12;11(1):189.

[33] Craiglow, B. G., Tavares, D., King, B. A. (2016). Topical Ruxolitinib for the Treatment of Alopecia Universalis. *JAMA Dermatol.* Apr; 152:490-1.

[34] Joshipura, D., Alomran, A., Zancanaro, P., Rosmarin, D. (2018). Treatment of vitiligo with the topical Janus kinase inhibitor ruxolitinib: A 32-week open-label extension study with optional narrow-bandultraviolet *B J Am Acad Dermatol.* Jun; 78(6):1205-1207.

In: Advances in Health and Disease
Editor: Lowell T. Duncan
ISBN: 978-1-53616-380-3

Chapter 5

Adverse Health Effects of Benzene Exposure in Children: Current Understandings and Perspectives

Mark A. D'Andrea, MD and G. Kesava Reddy*, PhD
University Cancer and Diagnostic Centers, Houston, TX, US

Abstract

Despite significant advances, the adverse health effects of benzene exposure in children have rarely been studied. Children at various developmental stages have unique physical risk factors when exposed to toxic chemicals such as benzene due to their levels of mobility, oxygen consumption, hormonal production, and overall growth. They are more susceptible to leukemogenesis because their hematopoietic cell populations are differentiating and undergoing maturation. The susceptibility to benzene may vary due to its effect that arises, in part, from genetic variations in its metabolism, DNA repair, genomic stability, and immune function. The pharmacokinetics of benzene differ widely between children and adults due to childrens' incomplete metabolic systems, rapid tissue regeneration, immature host defenses, activity

* Corresponding Author's Email: kreddy_usa@yahoo.com

patterns, and high rates of infection by respiratory pathogens. Thus, exposure to benzene can cause deleterious health effects among children. Given the importance of the toxicity of benzene, this chapter provides summaries of the current scientific knowledge and understanding of the clinical findings and health consequences of benzene exposure among children.

Abbreviations

ACQ = Asthma Control Questionnaire;
ALP = Alkaline phosphatase;
ALT = Alanine amino transferase;
AST = Aspartate amino transferase;
BP = British petroleum;
BUN = Blood urea nitrogen;
RBC = Red blood cells;
WBC = White blood cells.

Introduction

Benzene is a volatile aromatic hydrocarbon ubiquitously found in the environment [1]. It arises mostly from anthropogenic sources, notably combustion. Benzene is a natural component of both crude and refined petroleum and formed because of the incomplete combustion of fossil fuels such as petroleum products and coal [2]. It is also a component of tobacco smoke, gasoline, vehicle exhaust, and industrial emissions, and was used historically as an industrial solvent in industry and in consumer products [3]. The uses of benzene as a solvent are now restricted in many countries, but it is still produced in high volumes for use primarily as a chemical intermediate. Benzene ranks in the top 20 most abundantly produced chemicals in the United States and is a commercially important intermediate of many chemicals manufactured in the industry [4].

Over 98% of the benzene produced is derived from the petrochemical and petroleum refining industries [5]. Owing to its volatile properties, benzene is known as one of the main contributors to air pollutants in the environment [6]. As a contaminant, ambient benzene is found in the environment from both human activities and natural processes [7, 8]. As the primary pollutant of concern, the International Agency for Research on Cancer (IARC) has long been classified benzene as a carcinogen because it in fact causes leukemia and other malignancies in humans after their exposure to benzene [9].

HEALTH CONCERNS OF BENZENE EXPOSURE

Environmental benzene exposure is an important health concern. The human population at large can be exposed to benzene in polluted air and water and through the use of benzene-containing products. It has been clearly established that human exposure to benzene leads not only to malignant cancers [10, 11], but also to a wide range of adverse non-cancerous adverse health effects including functional aberration of respiratory, nervous, immune, hematological, hepatic, renal, cardio-vascular, and reproductive systems [12-17]. After its exposure, benzene is easily absorbed, widely distributed, and extensively metabolized, resulting in a complexity of reactive electrophiles through multiple metabolic pathways in various tissues, including the bone marrow. Following its absorption, benzene is metabolized by cytochrome P450 in the liver and forms active metabolites such as phenol, catechol, hydroquinone, and benzene oxide [18]. A schematic illustration of benzene's metabolism, its mechanisms of toxicity, and its toxic effects in humans is shown in Figure 1. These benzene metabolites suppress the immune system and leads to hematological toxicity, which is important not only as a health effect in its own right, but also as a biomarker and risk factor for leukemia [19, 20]. Additionally, benzene exposure induces oxidative DNA damage, DNA strand breaks, gene mutations, and micronuclei [20, 21]. Moreover, benzene can affect both B-cell and T-cell proliferation, reduce the host resistance to infection and produce chromosomal aberrations [22].

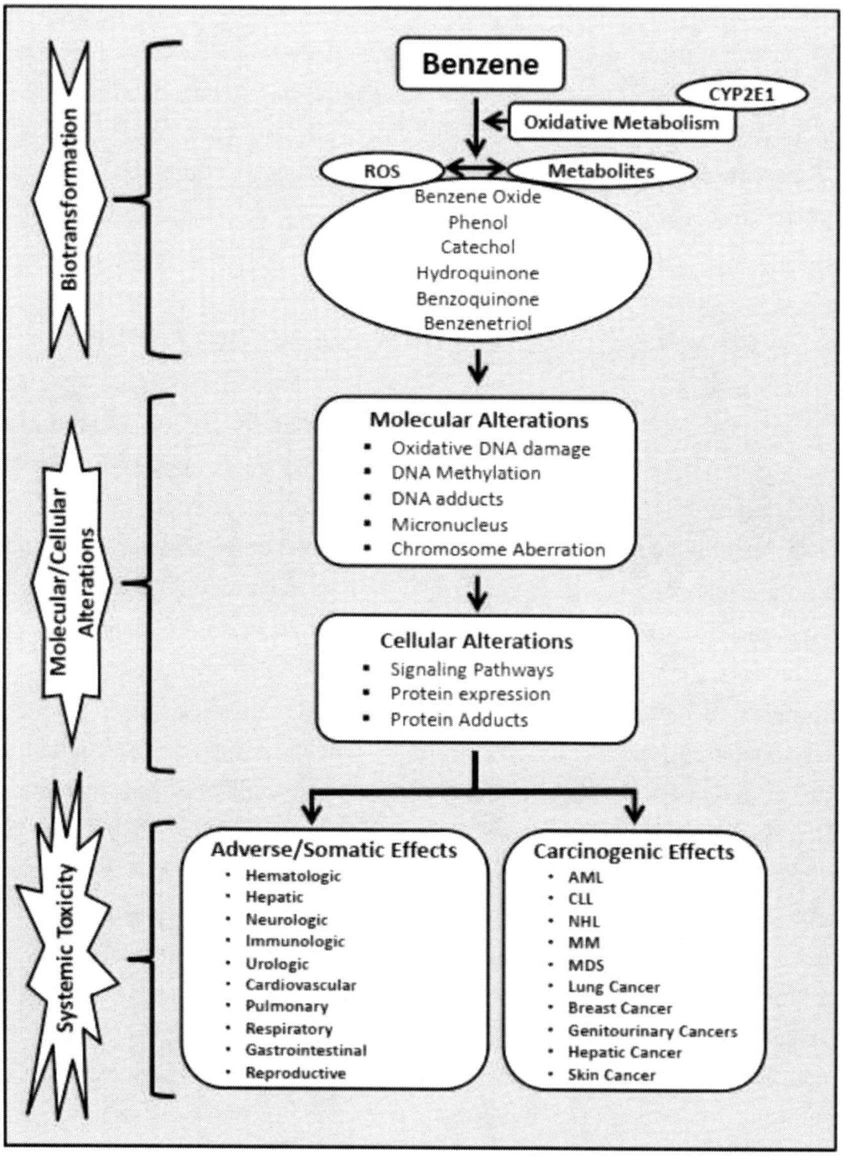

Figure 1. A schematic illustration of benzene metabolism, its mechanisms of toxicity, and its toxic effects in humans.

CHILDREN'S VULNERABILITY

The health effects of benzene exposure have been studied extensively in adults. Whereas, studies evaluating the health consequences of benzene exposure have rarely been reported in children. Emerging studies are demonstrating that benzene exposure can cause harmful health effects in children. Epidemiological studies suggest that benzene exposure is a major cause of childhood leukemia and other hematologic cancers [23-26]. The fact that children are growing and developing makes them more susceptible than adults to the adverse effects of environmental toxic pollutants. The higher susceptibility of children may be due to rapid growth and accompanying anatomical changes in various organs and organ systems, which critically differentiate children from adults. In addition, children are more sensitive than adults to the toxic effects of the chemicals due to their differences in physiology, immaturity of enzyme systems and clearance mechanisms [27-30]. Furthermore, children are more susceptible to leukemogenesis because their hematopoietic cell populations are differentiating and metabolic systems, immature host defenses, high rates of infection by respiratory pathogens [27, 28]. The activity patterns also make children more vulnerable to the toxic effects of benzene exposure. Moreover, the pharmacokinetics of benzene and its metabolites differs widely between children and adults. Given the importance of the toxic effects of the benzene, this chapter provides the current scientific knowledge and understanding of the clinical findings and health consequences of benzene exposure among children (Table 1).

Table 1. Summary of Studies on the effect of benzene exposure among children

Location of Study	Study Design	Childrens' Age	Sample Size	Observed Clinical Health Effects	Reference
Ulsan, Korea	Cohort	8-11 Years	192 (97 Benzene Exposed and 95 Control)	Reduced WBC, RBC, platelets, and lymphocytes counts, decreased hemoglobin in benzene exposed children compared with unexposed childrem	Lee et al. 2002 [31]

Table 1. (Continued)

Location of Study	Study Design	Childrens' Age	Sample Size	Observed Clinical Health Effects	Reference
Texas City, Texas, USA	Cohort	8-11 Years	312 (157 Benzene Exposed and 155 95 Control) children	Reduced WBC counts, increased platelet counts, elevated creatinine levels, and increased liver enzymes such as ALP, AST and ALT in benzene exposed children compared with unexposed children.	D'Andrea and Reddy 2014 [32]
Texas City, Texas, USA	Cohort	8-11 Years	899 (641 Benzene Exposed and 258 Control) children	Reduced WBC counts, increased platelet counts, decreased hemoglobin, hematocrit, and BUN levels, and increased liver enzymes such as ALP, AST and ALT in benzene exposed children compared with unexposed children.	D'Andrea and Reddy 2016 [33]
Four townships with 83 small villages on the west coast in the Republic of Korea	Cohort	5-16 Years	655 children	Exposure was associated with aggravation and persistence of asthma symptoms	Noh et al. 2019 [34]
Taean, The Republic of Korea	Cohort	Range: <9 Years to >12 Years	1361 children	Exposure was associated with significantly higher symptom risk of depression	Ha et al. 2013 [35]
Taean, The Republic of Korea	Cohort	6-12 Years	436 children	Significantly impaired lung function, increased prevalence of 'asthma, elevated bronchial hyper reactivity, and higher on-set of wheezing	Jung et al. 2013 [36]
Kanawha County, West Virginia, USA	Cohort	7-8 Years	7,796 children	Increased incidence of chronic respiratory symptoms in children attending schools located in a close proximity to chemical industries. Significant trends were observed for asthma-related responses such as a physician's diagnosis of asthma, persistent wheezing, and attacks of shortness of breath with wheezing in school children	Ware et al. 1993 [37]

Location of Study	Study Design	Childrens' Age	Sample Size	Observed Clinical Health Effects	Reference
				enrolled within a close proximity to chemical plants regions than those in the non-industrial region.	
La Plata, Argentina	Cohort	6-12 Years	1,191 (282 living close to the petro-chemical plants, 270 exposed to heavy traffic, and 639 living in non-polluted areas)	Significantly elevated asthma and respiratory symptoms including wheezing, cough, dyspnea, and rhinitis, and reduced lung function in children living near the petrochemical plant compared with those living in non-polluted areas.	Wichmann et al. 2009 [38]
Rio Grande do Norte, Brazil	Cross-sectional	0-14 Years	209 children	Higher incidence of respiratory symptoms in children exposed to petrochemicals	Moraes et al. 2010 [39]
El Paso, Texas, USA	Panel study	6-12 Years	36 children	Increased Asthma Control Questionnaire Score in children exposed to traffic pollution with benzene, toluene, and other toxins.	Zora et al. 2013 [40]
Asturias, Gipuzkoa, Sabadell, and Valencia, Spain	Cohort	12-18 Months	2,199 infants	Increased respiratory tract infections	Aguilera et al. 2013 [41]
Los Angeles, USA	Panel study	10-16 Years	21 children	Increased asthma and lung function among the children exposed to benzene	Delfino et al.2003 [42]
Viseu, Portugal	Panel study	6-8 Years	51 children	Deteriorated lung function in children exposed to benzene	Martins et al. 2012 [43]
Texas City, Texas, USA	Cohort	8-11 Years	312 (157 Benzene Exposed and 155 95 Control) children	Upper Respiratory (67%), neurological symptoms (57%), diarrhea (25%), cough (24%), dermatological (24%), nausea/vomiting (21%), gastrointestinal (12%), wheezing (9%), chest pain (6%), vision (6%), painful joints (6%), and urinary irritation (3%)	D'Andrea and Reddy 2016 [49]

WBC = White blood cells; RBC = Red blood cells; ALP = Alkaline phosphatase; AST = Aspartate amino transferase; ALT = Alanine amino transferase. BUN = Blood urea nitrogen.

Benzene Exposure and Alterations of Hematological Functions among Children

Alterations in hematological functions are not only relevant for diagnosing disorders of the hematological system but also helpful in the diagnosis of many organ and systemic diseases. A cohort study by Lee and coauthors [31] assessed the hematological changes in children living near vicinity of a petrochemical estate region in Ulsan, Korea, and who were environmentally exposed to volatile organic compounds containing low levels of benzene. This study included a total of 192 children between the ages of 8 years and 11 years who were living in close proximity to the petrochemical estate region or a suburban region of Ulsan, Korea. The exposed group was comprised of 48 boys and 49 girls who lived near the estate region and went to an elementary school located near the petrochemical site. The unexposed group was comprised of 46 boys and 49 girls who had lived in the suburban region 10 miles from the petrochemical estate region. Both the unexposed and benzene exposed groups had similar age and sex distributions. Hematological assessment revealed that, the total WBC counts and absolute lymphocytes counts of 11-year-old children living near the estate region were significantly lower than those of children living in the suburban region further away from the petrochemical site ($P = 0.009$, $P = 0.032$, respectively). Although the 8-year-old children living near the petrochemical estate region had decreased WBC counts and absolute lymphocytes counts compared with those living in the suburban region, they did not reach statistical significance. The RBC counts and hemoglobin levels of the 8-year-old exposed children were significantly lower than those of the unexposed children ($P < 0.001$, $P < 0.001$, respectively). A similar, but not statistically significant, trend was seen in the parameters of the 11-year-old exposed and unexposed groups. Whereas the platelet counts were significantly decreased in both the 8- and 11-year-old exposed children compared with those of the unexposed children (P-0.001, P-0.001, respectively). A follow up assessment at 3 and 6 months after their initial evaluation yielded similar differences but there were not consistent findings in the exposed and unexposed groups of the 8- and 11-year-old children.

The generalized linear model analysis of variance for the CBC values showed that the region where the exposure took place was a significant independent variable for the total WBC counts, RBC counts, and platelet counts ($P = 0.007$, $P = 0.004$, $P = 0.036$, respectively), and the childrens' sex was a significant independent variable for the RBC counts ($P = 0.001$). Similarly, age was a significant independent variable for the total WBC counts, absolute lymphocyte counts and platelet counts $P < 0.001$, $P = 0.004$, and $P = 0.005$, respectively). Overall, the study findings showed that environmental exposure to the volatile organic compounds containing low levels of benzene was associated clinically with a higher prevalence of hematological abnormalities in children living near the petrochemical estate region.

In a pilot study [32] we evaluated the hematological functions in children who were less than 17 years-old and exposed to benzene following BP's flaring incident in Texas City, Texas. A total of 312 children were included in the study. Of the 312 children, 157 were exposed to benzene and 155 were not exposed to benzene. Both unexposed and benzene exposed groups had similar age and sex distributions. Clinically, hematologic analysis showed that WBC counts were significantly decreased in the benzene exposed children compared with the unexposed children (P = 0.022). Conversely, the platelet counts were increased significantly in the benzene exposed group compared with the unexposed group (P = 0.005). Similarly, the serum creatinine levels were significantly increased in the benzene exposed children compared with the unexposed children (P = 0.000). However, no significant alterations were observed in the mean hemoglobin or hematocrit or BUN levels between the benzene exposed and unexposed children. The results of this pilot study indicated that environmental exposure to benzene was associated clinically with altered hematological profiles in those children who were exposed to benzene from the flaring incident at the BP refinery facility in Texas City, Texas.

In a larger cohort study, we further assessed the hematological changes that occured in children exposed to benzene following the flaring incident [33]. A total of 899 children aged < 17 years were included in the study. Of the 899 children, 258 were unexposed and 641 were exposed to benzene. The mean age of the unexposed and exposed children was 10.5 and 9.5 years, respectively. Among the unexposed children, there were 57% male and 43% female children. In the benzene exposed group, there were 52%males and 48% females.

Hematological analysis indicated that those children exposed to benzene had significantly decreased mean WBC counts compared with those of the unexposed children (P = 0.001). Conversely, the mean platelet counts in the benzene exposed group were significantly higher when compared with those of the unexposed children group (P = 0.001). Whereas the mean hemoglobin levels decreased significantly in the benzene exposed group compared with those of the unexposed group P = 0.001). Similarly, the percentage of hematocrit decreased significantly among the benzene exposed children compared with those of the unexposed children (P = 0.001). BUN was also found to be reduced significantly in the benzene exposed group compared with those of the unexposed group (P = 0.001). However, no significant differences were noted in the serum creatinine levels between the benzene exposed and unexposed groups. Furthermore, sub-analysis indicated that, regardless of age or gender, significant alterations in the hematological profiles were seen in those children exposed to benzene. Overall, the findings of the hematological profiles confirmed the pilot study findings indicating that children who have been exposed to benzene have significantly increased health risks compared to unexposed children.

BENZENE EXPOSURE AND ALTERATIONS OF HEPATIC FUNCTION AMONG CHILDREN

The liver is the principal organ of xenobiotic metabolism and hence it is very important to monitor its function in people exposed to benzene or other toxins. It is well known that phosphatases, amino transferases, and dehydrogenases are important enzymes in biological processes. They are involved in the detoxification, metabolism and biosynthesis of energetic macromolecules for different essential functions. Any interference in these enzymes leads to biochemical impairment and lesions in the tissue and cellular function. Thus, the measurement of these liver enzyme such as ALP, AST and ALT are routinely assessed as indicators for hepatic dysfunction and damage.

Currently, there are no published studies in literature that have evaluated the harmful effects of benzene exposure on the liver functions in children except the research work published by the authors [32, 33]. The initial pilot study included 157 benzene exposed and 155 unexposed children and assessed their liver function enzymes such as alkaline phosphatase (ALP), aspartate amino transferase (AST), and alanine amino transferase (ALT). The study findings revealed that benzene exposed children had clinically significantly higher levels of ALP ($P = 0.04$), AST ($P = 0.015$), and ALT ($P = 0.005$) compared with the unexposed children.

Subsequently, the larger cohort study [33] assessed the liver function enzymes in 641 benzene exposed children and compared with the 258 unexposed children. Serum ALP, AST and ALT levels were reported to be increased significantly in children exposed to benzene compared with the unexposed children ($P = 0.001$). Furthermore, sub-group analysis indicated that, regardless of age or gender, significant alterations in hepatic enzymes were seen in those children exposed to benzene. Overall, the findings of the hepatic profiles confirmed the pilot study findings indicating that children who have been exposed to benzene have significantly increased health risks compared to unexposed children.

BENZENE EXPOSURE AND ILLNESS SYMPTOMS AMONG CHILDREN

Among all, respiratory illness symptoms are the most often studied health complaints in children exposed to either benzene or oil spill or petrochemicals or urban traffic pollutants. Upper respiratory symptoms were the most frequently reported followed by other illness symptoms. Other illness symptoms included neurological symptoms, cough, and shortness of breath, chest tightness and vision difficulty.

It is well known that crude oil is mixture of multiple volatile organic compounds including benzene, toluene ethylbenzene, xylene and other toxic chemicals. Following oil spill, these toxic chemicals pollute surroundings and persist in various environmental media and bioaccumulate over the long-term. Noh and colleagues [34] recently assessed the long-term effect of the Hebei Spirit's oil spill in 655 middle school children. Specifically, the investigators assessed children's asthma symptoms using survey questionnaire at one year (n = 655), three years (n = 664), and five years (n = 611) after their exposure to oil spill following the accident. A significant longitudinal relationship was seen between oil spill exposure and asthma symptoms in children. Specifically the study found oil spill exposure was associated with aggravation and persistence of asthma symptoms from cross-sectional and longitudinal observations up to five years after the accident. In addition, an increase in the prevalence of asthma symptoms was observed at one year, three years, and five years after the oil spill suggesting long-lasting and perhaps irreversible airway damage in children following their exposure to toxic chemical of the oil spill.

The mental health effects of the *Hebei Spirit* oil spill were assessed by Ha et al. [35] in schoolchildren living in the affected area, where most of their families were victims of the disaster. The investigators divided the child population according to distance of school they attended from the contaminated coastline. A cross-sectional questionnaire survey was conducted using the Children's Depression Inventory and State Anxiety Inventory in children attending elementary schools in the affected area. The information on distances between the nearest contaminated coastline to the child's residential house or attending school were obtained using a web-based map by inputting two address points. Of the 1,467 children who responded to the questionnaire at baseline, 1,361 were included in the analysis. The study showed that children whose schools were located closest to the contaminated coastline had a significantly higher symptom risk of depression compared to those who lived farthest from the affected areas (odds ratio [OR], 2.73; 95% confidence interval, 1.40 - 5.33). However, no significant association was seen between anxiety symptoms and distance.

Jung and colleagues [36] evaluated the respiratory effects in schoolchildren who lived along the affected area of the *Hebei Spirit* oil spill. Of 662 children living in the area exposed to the oil spill, 436 were participated as subjects. The Modified International Study of Asthma and Allergies in Childhood questionnaire was used to evaluate characteristics related to asthma. The findings of the study revealed that children who lived close to the oil spill area showed a significantly impaired lung function, increased prevalence of 'asthma, elevated prevalence of bronchial hyper reactivity, and higher on-set of wheezing compared to those who resided far from the oil spill area. Collectively, the study findings suggest that oil spill exposure is a risk factor for asthma in children.

A study by Ware and co-investigators [37] evaluated the respiratory and irritant health effects of ambient volatile organic compounds in 7,796 children attending 74 elementary schools located in chemical industry regions. The findings indicated that exposure to volatile organic compounds from chemical manufacturing plants was associated with an increased incidence of chronic respiratory symptoms in children attending schools located in a close proximity to the chemical industries. Significant trends were observed for asthma-related responses such as a physician's diagnosis of asthma, persistent wheezing, and attacks of shortness of breath with wheezing in school children enrolled within a close proximity to regions containing chemical plants than those in the non-industrial regions.

Similar findings were reported in a study by Wichmann et al. [38] that assessed the effects of exposure to petrochemical pollution on the respiratory health of children aged 6 to 12 years living close to petrochemical plants (n = 282) and compared them with those living in a region with exposure to heavy traffic (n = 270) or in relatively non-polluted areas (n = 639) in La Plata, Argentina. The findings showed that children living near the petrochemical plant had significantly elevated asthma and respiratory symptoms (wheezing, cough, dyspnea, and rhinitis) and significantly reduced lung functions than those living in non-polluted regions ($P < 0.001$). Moraes and coworkers [39] investigated the health impacts of living near petrochemical plants by assessing respiratory illnesses in 209 Brazilian children. The results from this study revealed that respiratory symptoms were found to be increased in children among communities in the vicinity of a petrochemical complex particularly those living downwind from the plant.

A panel study conducted by Zora et al. [40] assessed the associations between urban air pollution of benzene and pediatric asthma control using an Asthma Control Questionnaire (ACQ) score in two elementary schools located in high and low traffic areas of El Paso, Texas. Eligibility criteria included age of the children between 6 and 12 years, a physician diagnosis of asthma, no other lung disease or major illness, a non-smoking household, and residence proximal to their school. Data was reported for 36 of the 38 children who completed the protocol. The study found that benzene levels in the air of a school located in high traffic area ranged from 0.2 to 2.4 $\mu g/m^3$. Although no significant associations between benzene and other pollutants with an increase in ACQ score were found, an increase in ACQ score was related with an increase in benzene levels among children inhaling corticosteroids daily. Aguilera et al. [41] investigated the association of air pollution exposure during pregnancy and respiratory illnesses, ear infections, and eczema during the first 12–18 months of life in a Spanish birth cohort of 2,199 infants. These authors observed that during the second trimester of pregnancy, an increase in 1.0 $\mu g/m^3$ of benzene exposure was associated with an increased risk of lower respiratory tract infections in those infants.

In a panel study, Delfino et al. [42] examined the longitudinal relationship of the daily asthma severity among asthmatic children exposed to volatile organic compounds such as benzene. The study included 21 asthmatic children between 10-16 years of age. The study revealed that increased mean concentrations of benzene (5.7$\mu g/m^3$) levels were associated with increased asthma and poor lung function among the children. Martins and co-authors [43] evaluated the relationship between air polluted by benzene exposure and airway changes in a group of wheezing children. The investigators included a total of 51 wheezing children with a mean age 7.3 years from Viseu, Portugal. Benzene levels were monitored for 4 weeks and using a dispersion model, personal exposure was determined based on time-activity patterns according to the estimations. These authors reported that an increase in 10.0 $\mu g/m^3$ of benzene exposure was associated with deteriorated lung function-related outcomes in wheezing children.

In a pilot study, we investigated the clinical presentation of the illness symptoms experienced by children who were exposed to benzene following a flaring incident at the BP refinery in Texas City, Texas [32]. The study included a total of 157 children who were exposed to benzene. Among the illness symptoms, neurological symptoms such as unsteady gait, memory loss, and headaches were the most (80%) frequently reported symptoms in children exposed to benzene. Upper respiratory symptoms were reported by 48% of the benzene exposed children followed by cough (48%), nausea/vomiting (43%), dermatological (36%), shortness of breath (32%), wheezing (27%), dizziness (22%), chest pain (15%), painful joints (15%), and weight loss (13%). To complement these findings, recently we conducted a full-fledged study in 641 children (n = 641) who were exposed to benzene following a flaring incident at the BP refinery in Texas City, Texas [44]. A total of 1,790 illness symptoms were observed in 641 children exposed to benzene.

Among all clinically presented illness symptoms, upper respiratory symptoms occurred as the most frequently (67%) followed by neurological symptoms (57%), diarrhea (25%), and cough (24%). Logistic regression analysis indicated that neurological symptoms (R^2 = 0.75), chest pain (R^2 = 0.64), joint pain (R^2 = 0.57), vision difficulty (R^2 = 0.54) were positively associated with increasing age of the children. Overall, the findings revealed that children exposed to benzene experienced a range of illness symptoms indicating their vulnerability to increased risks and health complications to benzene exposure.

Clinical Implications

Clinical evidence suggests that hemotoxicity is the major effect and is unique to benzene. Exposure to benzene causes bone marrow injury resulting in hemotoxicity leading to changes in white blood cells, platelets, hemoglobin, hematocrit, and other blood cells formation. Multiple mechanisms including alterations in the expression of numerous genes and proteins, DNA methylation patterns, and RNA profiles appear to play an important role in benzene induced hemotoxicity in exposed children [45].

Although several studies have investigated the effect of benzene exposure on the hematological changes in adults, only a handful of studies published so far have evaluated the clinical changes in the hematological functions among children following their exposure to benzene [31-33]. The findings of these studies demonstrate that children exposed to benzene experienced significantly reduced hematological indices compared with those of unexposed children. However, conflicting findings in platelet counts were observed in the benzene exposed children. Our recently published studies demonstrated significantly elevated platelet counts in children who were exposed to benzene compared with unexposed children [32, 33]. However, in the study reported by Lee and associates [31] significantly decreased platelet counts were observed in children exposed to benzene compared with those of unexposed children. Although the discrepancies in the platelet counts in benzene exposed children currently cannot fully explained, Ceresa and coworkers [46] have found that thrombocytopenia was not a constant finding in most of the adult subjects who were exposed to benzene. Nevertheless, additional studies are warranted to clarify the effect of benzene exposure on the platelet counts in children.

The liver is the principal organ of xenobiotic metabolism and hence it is very important to monitor its function in people exposed to benzene or other toxins. It is well known that phosphatases, amino transferases, and dehydrogenases are important enzymes in biological processes. They are involved in the detoxification, metabolism and biosynthesis of energetic macromolecules for different essential functions. Any interference in these enzymes leads to biochemical impairment and lesions in the tissue and altered cellular function. Thus, the measurement of these liver enzyme such as ALP, AST and ALT are routinely used as indicators for hepatic dysfunction and damage [47, 48]. In normal conditions, these enzymes are confined to the cells and are released into circulating blood when there is a necrosis or hepatic injury. Despite its importance, until recently, there were no published studies available in the literature evaluating the effect of benzene exposure on the hepatic functions in children. The two recent studies reported by the authors [32, 33] revealed that the serum levels of ALP, AST and ALT were found to be elevated among those children who were exposed to benzene indicating hepatic abnormalities in these children. The increase in the levels of these liver enzymes in their serum suggests the impairment or damage of the hepatic functions in children exposed to benzene.

Studies assessing the somatic or clinically presenting illness symptoms such as the respiratory, neurological, gastrointestinal, and other symptoms in children exposed to benzene are also limited in published literature. However, evidence from available studies suggests that benzene exposure is associated clinically with increased illness symptoms in children. The most common clinical presentation of these illness symptoms include those involving neurological and respiratory symptoms with shortness of breath, wheezing, dizziness, chest pain, and painful joints.

CONCLUSION

Together, studies evaluating the clinical changes in the hematologic, cardiac, hepatic, renal, and other vital organ functions in children who were exposed to benzene are sparse. We have yet to learn and to understand the full extent of all the adverse effects that benzene exposure has on pediatric populations. Findings from the currently available literature reveal that benzene exposure is associated with clinical abnormalities in the hematologic, hepatic, respiratory, and pulmonary functions in children. The hematological abnormalities were characterized by changes in RBC, WBC, absolute lymphocytes, platelets, hemoglobin, hematocrit and creatinine in benzene exposed children. Similarly, the hepatic abnormalities were characterized by elevated levels of ALP, AST and ALT enzymes in the serum of the children exposed to benzene. Few studies have evaluated the somatic or illness symptoms such as respiratory, neurological, gastrointestinal, and other symptoms in children exposed to benzene. Together these findings indicate that exposure to benzene may lead to clinically detectable detrimental health effects in children. However, to fully understand the importance and nature of these effects, further longitudinal and mechanistic studies on the health effects of benzene exposure in children are warranted.

Financial Disclosure

The authors have no financial relationships relevant to this article to disclose.

References

[1] Fenga C, Gangemi S, Costa C. Benzene exposure is associated with epigenetic changes (Review). *Mol Med Rep* 2016;13:3401-5.

[2] Duarte-Davidson R, Courage C, Rushton L, et al. Benzene in the environment: an assessment of the potential risks to the health of the population. *Occup Environ Med* 2001;58:2-13.

[3] Wallace L. Environmental exposure to benzene: an update. *Environ Health Perspect* 1996;104 Suppl 6:1129-36.

[4] Kirschner EM. Production of top 50 chemicals increased substantially in 1994 *Chem Eng News* 1995;73:16-20.

[5] OSHA. Occupational exposure to benzene. Final Rule.U.S. Department of Labor, Occupational Safety and Health Administration. *Fed Regist* 1987;52:34460–34578.

[6] Bahadar H, Mostafalou S, Abdollahi M. Current understandings and perspectives on non-cancer health effects of benzene: a global concern. Toxicol Appl Pharmacol 2014;276:83-94.

[7] Kotb MA, Ramadan HS, Shams El-Din R, et al. Changes in some biophysical and biochemical parameters in blood and urine of workers chronically exposed to benzene. *European Scientific Journal* 2013;9:411-422.

[8] Reynolds P, Von Behren J, Gunier RB, et al. Traffic patterns and childhood cancer incidence rates in California, United States. *Cancer Causes Control* 2002;13:665-73.

[9] IARC. Chemicals and industrial processes associated with cancer in humans: an updating of IARC monographs. *IARC Monogr Eval Carcinog Risks Hum. Volume 1 to 20.* suppl 1: 15., 1979.

[10] Costantini AS, Benvenuti A, Vineis P, et al. Risk of leukemia and multiple myeloma associated with exposure to benzene and other organic solvents: evidence from the Italian Multicenter Case-control study. *Am J Ind Med* 2008;51:803-11.

[11] Khalade A, Jaakkola MS, Pukkala E, et al. Exposure to benzene at work and the risk of leukemia: a systematic review and meta-analysis. *Environ Health* 2010;9:31.

[12] Bahadar H, Mostafalou S, Abdollahi M. Current understandings and perspectives on non-cancer health effects of benzene: a global concern. *Toxicol Appl Pharmacol* 2014;276:83-94.

[13] Baslo A, Aksoy M. Neurological abnormalities in chronic benzene poisoning. A study of six patients with aplastic anemia and two with preleukemia. *Environ Res* 1982;27:457-65.

[14] Dere E, Ari F. Effect of Benzene on liver functions in rats (Rattus norvegicus). *Environ Monit Assess* 2009;154:23-7.

[15] Dundarz MR, Turkbay T, Akay C, et al. Antioxidant enzymes and lipid peroxidation in adolescents with inhalant abuse. *Turk J Pediatr* 2003;45:43-5.

[16] Kotseva K, Popov T. Study of the cardiovascular effects of occupational exposure to organic solvents. *Int Arch Occup Environ Health* 1998;71 Suppl:S87-91.

[17] Mandiracioglu A, Akgur S, Kocabiyik N, et al. Evaluation of neuropsychological symptoms and exposure to benzene, toluene and xylene among two different furniture worker groups in Izmir. *Toxicol Ind Health* 2011;27:802-9.

[18] Gut I, Nedelcheva V, Soucek P, et al. Cytochromes P450 in benzene metabolism and involvement of their metabolites and reactive oxygen species in toxicity. *Environ Health Perspect* 1996;104 Suppl 6:1211-8.

[19] McHale CM, Zhang L, Smith MT. Current understanding of the mechanism of benzene-induced leukemia in humans: implications for risk assessment. *Carcinogenesis* 2012;33:240-52.

[20] Smith MT. Advances in understanding benzene health effects and susceptibility. *Annu Rev Public Health* 2010;31:133-48

[21] Barreto G, Madureira D, Capani F, et al. The role of catechols and free radicals in benzene toxicity: an oxidative DNA damage pathway. *Environ Mol Mutagen* 2009;50:771-80.

[22] Minciullo PL, Navarra M, Calapai G, et al. Cytokine network involvement in subjects exposed to benzene. *J Immunol Res* 2014;2014:937987.

[23] Vinceti M, Rothman KJ, Crespi CM, et al. Leukemia risk in children exposed to benzene and PM10 from vehicular traffic: a case-control study in an Italian population. *Eur J Epidemiol* 2012;27:781-90.

[24] Heck JE, Wu J, Lombardi C, et al. Childhood cancer and traffic-related air pollution exposure in pregnancy and early life. *Environ Health Perspect* 2013;121:1385-91.

[25] Freedman DM, Stewart P, Kleinerman RA, et al. Household solvent exposures and childhood acute lymphoblastic leukemia. *Am J Public Health* 2001;91:564-7.

[26] Pyatt D, Hays S. A review of the potential association between childhood leukemia and benzene. *Chem Biol Interact* 2010;184:151-64.

[27] Whitworth KW, Symanski E, Coker AL. Childhood lymphohematopoietic cancer incidence and hazardous air pollutants

in southeast Texas, 1995-2004. *Environ Health Perspect* 2008; 116:1576-80.

[28] Goldman, L. R. Children--unique and vulnerable. Environmental risks facing children and recommendations for response. *Environ Health Perspect* 1995;103 Suppl 6:13-8.

[29] Bearer, C. F. How are children different from adults? *Environ Health Perspect* 1995;103 Suppl 6:7-12.

[30] Bearer, C. F. Environmental health hazards: how children are different from adults. *Future Child* 1995;5:11-26.

[31] Lee, C. R., Yoo, C. I., Lee, J. H., et al. Hematological changes of children exposed to volatile organic compounds containing low levels of benzene. *Sci Total Environ* 2002;299:237-45.

[32] D'Andrea, M. A., Reddy, G. K. Health effects of benzene exposure among children following a flaring incident at the British Petroleum Refinery in Texas City. *Pediatr Hematol Oncol* 2014;31:1-10.

[33] D'Andrea, M. A., Reddy, G. K. Adverse Health Effects of Benzene Exposure Among Children Following a Flaring Incident at the British Petroleum Refinery in Texas City. *Clin Pediatr (Phila)* 2016;55:219-27.

[34] Noh S. R., Kim J. A., Cheong H. K., et al. Hebei Spirit oil spill and its long-term effect on children's asthma symptoms. *Environ Pollut* 2019;248:286-294.

[35] Ha, M., Jeong, W. C., Lim, M., et al. Children's Mental Health in the Area Affected by the Hebei Spirit Oil Spill Accident. *Environ Health Toxicol* 2013;28:e2013010.

[36] Jung, S. C., Kim, K. M., Lee, K. S., et al. Respiratory effects of the hebei spirit oil spill on children in taean, Korea. *Allergy Asthma Immunol* Res 2013;5:365-70.

[37] Ware, J. H., Spengler, J. D., Neas, L. M., et al. Respiratory and irritant health effects of ambient volatile organic compounds. The Kanawha County Health Study. *Am J Epidemiol* 1993;137:1287-301.

[38] Wichmann F. A., Muller, A., Busi, L. E., et al. Increased asthma and respiratory symptoms in children exposed to petrochemical pollution. *J Allergy Clin Immunol* 2009;123:632-8.

[39] Moraes, A. C., Ignotti, E., Netto, P.A., et al. Wheezing in children and adolescents living next to a petrochemical plant in Rio Grande do Norte, *Brazil. J Pediatr (Rio J)* 2010;86:337-44.

[40] Zora, J. E., Sarnat, S. E., Raysoni, A. U., et al. Associations between urban air pollution and pediatric asthma control in El Paso, *Texas. Sci Total Environ* 2013;448:56-65.

[41] Aguilera, I., Pedersen, M., Garcia-Esteban, R., et al. Early-life exposure to outdoor air pollution and respiratory health, ear infections, and eczema in infants from the INMA study. *Environ Health Perspect* 2013;121:387-92.

[42] Delfino, R. J., Gong, H., Linn, W. S., et al. Respiratory symptoms and peak expiratory flow in children with asthma in relation to volatile organic compounds in exhaled breath and ambient air. *J Expo Anal Environ Epidemiol* 2003;13:348-63.

[43] Martins, P. C., Valente, J., Papoila, A. L., et al. Airways changes related to air pollution exposure in wheezing children. *Eur Respir J* 2012;39:246-53.

[44] D'Andrea, M. A., Reddy, G. K. Adverse Health Complaints of Adults Exposed to Benzene After a Flaring Disaster at the BP Refinery Facility in Texas City, Texas. *Disaster Med Public Health Prep* 2017:1-9.

[45] Zhang, L., McHale, C. M., Rothman, N., et al. Systems biology of human benzene exposure. *Chem Biol Interact* 2010;184:86-93.

[46] Ceresa, C., Grazioli, C., Monteverde, A. [On the behavior of thromboelastograms in rice-field leptospirosis]. *Minerva Med* 1960;51:3544-52.

[47] Khan, I. A., Reddy, B. V., Mahboob, M., et al. Effects of phosphorothionate on the reproductive system of male rats. J. *Environ. Sci. Health Part B* 2001;36:445-456.

[48] Innerfield, F. *Enzymes in clinical chemistry New York*, USA.: McGraw Hill Publications, 1960.

In: Advances in Health and Disease
Editor: Lowell T. Duncan
ISBN: 978-1-53616-380-3

Chapter 6

PREDICTION OF AQUATIC TOXICITY IN PIMEPHALES PROMELAS OF SUBSTITUTED BENZENES IN SILICO METHODOLOGIES

Nadia Ziani[1,*], Khadidja Amirat[1] and Djelloul Messadi[1]
[1]Environmental and Food Safety Laboratory, Faculty of Science,
Badji Mokhtar University Annaba,
Annaba, Algeria

ABSTRACT

Benzene, a monocyclic aromatic hydrocarbon, is a carcinogenic liquid. Before the 1920s, benzene was frequently used as an industrial solvent, particularly for degreasing metals. When its toxicity becomes obvious, it is replaced by other solvents for applications requiring direct exposure of the user. Benzene is used for the most part as an intermediate in the synthesis of other chemical compounds. A hybrid [Genetic algorithm (GA/Artificial neural network (ANN)] QSAR model was

* Corresponding Author's Email: ziani_nadia84@yahoo.fr.

developed for the prediction of aqueous toxicity. The data concerning 92 substituted benzenes was separated into two disjoined subsets, respectively 74 elements for calculating and testing of the model, and 18 elements for its external validation. Theoretical molecular descriptors were calculated by using commercially available software of molecular modeling. The size of the model was determined by optimizing the FIT of KUBINYI, and the selection of the descriptors realized by genetic algorithm. The values of the statistical parameters (R^2, Q^2, Q^2ext, SDEC, SDEP, SDEPext) obtained attest relevance of the developed model.

Keywords: Substituted Benzenes, Aquatic Toxicity, Theoretical Molecular Descriptors, Hybrid GA/ANN model

1. Introduction

Substituted benzenes, which have considerable industrial and commercial importance, are extensively used for the production of isocyanides, dyes, and agricultural and pharmaceutical products (Lin and Juang 2009) [1].

The ecological risk assessment (ERA) of chemicals is a necessary measure to control and prevent the risks of chemicals to the aquatic species. The chronic toxicity of aquatic species is an indispensable biological endpoint for the ERA (VanLeeuwen and Vermeire 2007) [2]. In order to assess the ecological risk of chemicals, the information on aquatic toxicity is required [3] (Hodges et al. 2006).

REACH regulation demands information about acute toxicity of chemicals towards fish and supports the use of QSAR models, provided compliance with OECD principles. Existing models present some drawbacks that may limit their regulatory application. Among the latter methods, quantitative structure–activity relationship's (QSAR) analysis emerged as one of the suggested approaches because of its low cost and time for application.

QSAR analysis comprises a variety of mathematical and statistical methods that aim at finding functional relationships between the structures of chemical compounds described by means of experimental or theoretical variables called molecular descriptors [4] and their measured properties and activities.

This study focuses on the development of a new (Quantitative structure activity relationship (QSAR) model to predict the acute toxicity of diverse chemicals, defined as LC50 96 hours, towards the fathead minnow (Pimephales promelas). The model was developed the five OECD principles kept in mind in order to make it applicable for regulatory purposes within REACH. To this end, attention was paid to the curation of the experimental data, which led to the definition of an extended dataset consisting of 92 organic molecules. The model, based on six molecular descriptors, used a similarity-based algorithm (kNN) to predict the toxicity. The applicability domain (AD) was automatically evaluated for each prediction and an additional analysis of the performance was carried out for individual functional groups. The predictive power was estimated by means of thorough and appropriate internal and external validation procedures.

Moreover, the chemical information encoded by model descriptors was explained, and we attempted to put it in relation with aquatic toxicity. Eventually, an example of the application of the model was given.

2. METHODES

The QSPR study of these benzenes and related derivate compounds was performed with the selection of the data set, generation of molecular descriptors, multiple linear regression statistical analysis and model validation techniques.

2.1. Experimental Data

The known experimental pCL50 values for a diverse data set consisting of benzenes and related derivates compounds was taken from literature [5] (Kier and Hall 1986).

2.2. Calculation and Selection of Descriptors

The chemical structure of each compound was sketched on a PC using the HYPERCHEM Program [6] (HYPERCHEM software 2002) and pre-optimized using the MM+ molecular mechanics method (Polak-Ribiere algorithm). The final geometries of the minimum energy conformation were obtained by the semi-empirical PM3 method at a restricted Hartree-Fock level with no configuration interaction and an application of a gradient norm limit of 0.001kcal·A^{-1}·mol^{-1} as a stopping criterion. Then, the geometries were used as input for the generation of 1664 descriptors using the Dragon software (Version 5.4) [7] (Todeschini et al. 2005). The selection of a minimum set of significant descriptors was carried out by genetic algorithm in the MOBYDIGS [8] version of Todeschini maximizing R^2, Q^2_{LOO} and Q^2_{ext}.

The size of the model is fixed by optimizing the value of the KUBINYI FIT function [9], which was calculated according to (1):

$$FIT=\frac{R^2}{1-R^2}\frac{n-p-1}{(n+p)^2} \quad (1)$$

2.3. Chemometric Methods

2.3.1. Multiple Linear Regression

MLR is a statistical tool that regresses independent variables against a dependent variable. The objective of MLR is to find a linear model of the property of interest, which takes the form below:

$$Y= a_0+\sum_{i=1}^{n} a_i x_i \quad (2)$$

where: y: is the property, which is, the dependent variable

x_i: represent molecular descriptors.

a_i: represent the coefficients of those descriptors and a_0 is the intercept of the equation.

2.3.2. Artificial Neural Networks

Artificial neural networks (ANN) are artificial systems simulating the function of the human brain. Three components constitute a neural network: the processing elements or nodes, the topology of the connections between the nodes, and the learning rule by which new information is encoded in the network. While there are a number of different artificial neural networks models, the most frequently used type of Artificial Neural Networks in QSAR is the three-layered feed-forward network (Zupan and Gasteiger 1993). In this type of network, the neurons are arranged in layers (an input layer, one hidden layer and an output layer). Each neuron in any layer is fully connected with the neurons of a succeeding layer and there are no connections between neurons belonging to the same layer.

3. RESULTS AND DISCUSSION

3.1. Models Calculation

The graph of the figure reproduces the variations of the FIT (eq.1) according to the number of variables of the model. It is obvious that the optimum model (maximum FIT) has 4 variables.

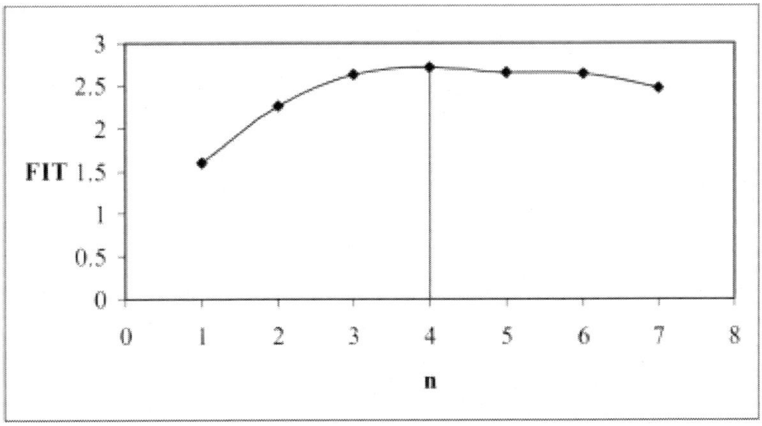

Figure 1. Variation of the Fit according to the number of descriptors.

Table 1. Molecular descriptors involved in the modeling of lethal concentration 50

No	Symbol	Class	Meaning
1	MAXDP	Topological Descriptors	Positive electrotropic variation Max.
2	X5Av	Connectivity index	Valances connectivity index average chi-5
3	HTp	GETAWAY descriptors	Total index H / weighted by Atomic polarizabilities
4	R6e	GETAWAY descriptors	Autocorrelation R of lag 6 / weighted by atomic electronegativities of Sanderson.

Both methods (MLR, ANN) were used to predict the lethal concentration of 50 out of 92 benzene derivatives. Thus, the results obtained will be compared. The following graph optimizes the size of the model. The four explanatory variables used for the two methods are summarized in Table 1.

3.2. Optimization by Artificial Neural Networks (ANN)

Using these descriptors for neural optimization, and after looking for the number of neurons in the hidden layer, the learning algorithm used is Retro propagation of the error gradient.

3.3. Calculation of Models (MLR and ANN)

In the case of the MLR, the four-variable model is:

$$pLC = 1.06 + 0.274\ MAXDP + 25.5\ X5Av + 0.401\ HTp - 0.557\ R6u \quad (3)$$

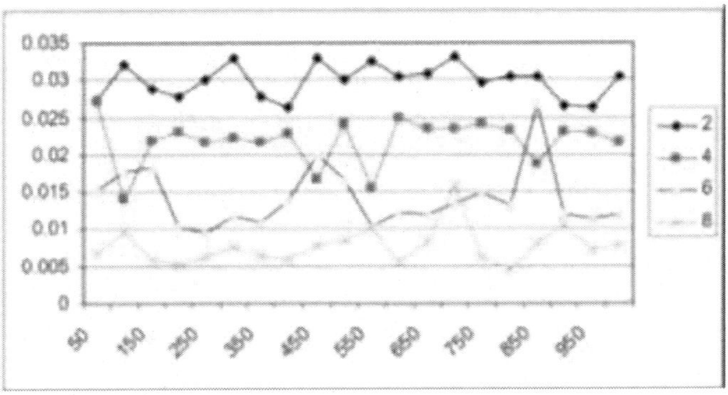

Figure 2. selection of the number of neurons of the hidden layer.

Table 2. Optimal structure of the neural network

Number of inputs	**4 (the descriptors)**
Number of outputs	01 (The lethal concentration 50)
Number of hidden layers	01
Number of neurons in the hidden layer	06
Learning Algorithm	Retro propagation of the error gradient
Learning functions	Hyperbolic tangent

In the case of the RNA, the selection of the number of neurons of the hidden layer is fixed at six (06). The following graph explains this choice.

3.4. Analysis and Comparison of Results

The residue analysis shows, for the MLR, a mean absolute error equal to 0.23, and two observations: 33 and 79 with errors greater than 3s = 0.92.

On the other hand, the ANN presents an absolute average error of 0.11. There were also three observations, 77, 78 and 87, that have an error greater than 0.399 (3s).

Table 3. Values of the statistical parameters for the test set

	MLR	ANN
n	92	92
R^2	78.77	95.69
σ_N	0.315	0.15
Q^2	76.04	94.91
F	64	363.798

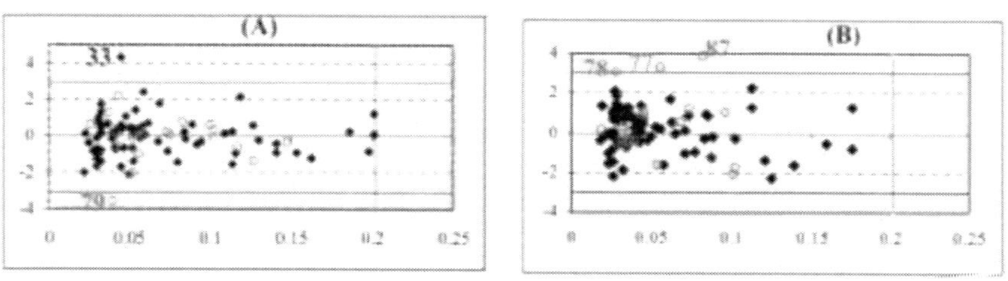

Figure 3. Williams Diagram. (A): MLR; (B): ANN.

Table 3, which groups together other statistical parameters, highlights the best results obtained by exploiting a nonlinear correlation (ANN).

Williams's diagrams for the multilinear (A) and nonlinear (B) regressions are reproduced in Figure 3. They show two outliers for the MLR (33 and 79) and three for the ANN (77; 78 and 87).

The quality of the fit was checked each time by cross-validation with "leave -one-out". (Figure 4).

The Q^2_{LOO} factor values (Figure 4) show the best stability presented by the nonlinear model (ANN).

pLC50= 0.164315 + 0.962515 Y-Pred

pLC50= 0.164315 + 0.962515 Y-Pred

S = 0.330571; R^2= 74.7%; R^2 (adjusted) = 74.4%

S = 0.645404; R^2= 99.5%; R^2 (adjusted) = 99.5%

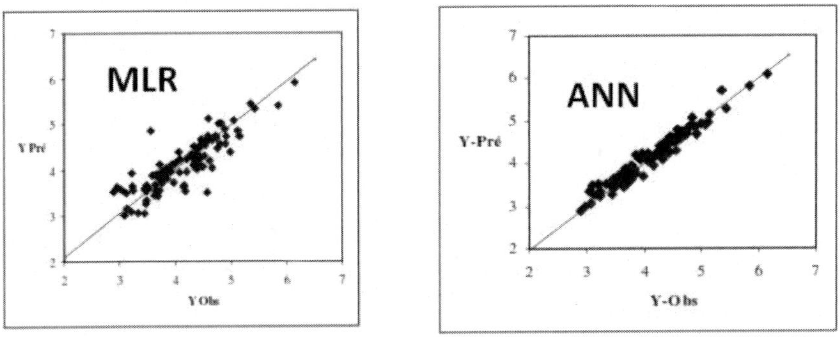

Figure 4. Graph of the predicted pCL50 (i) values according to the observed values.

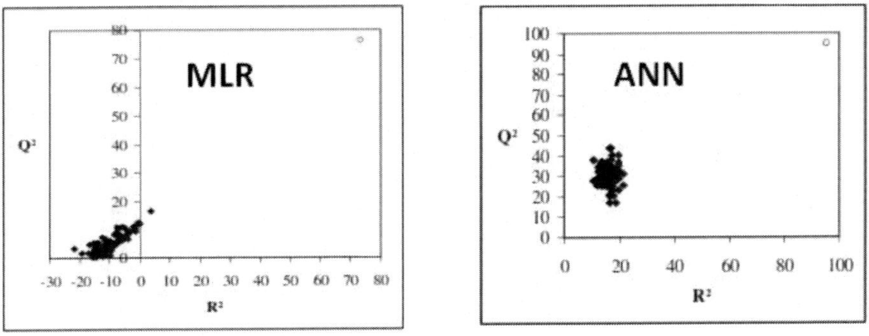

Figure 5. Randomization Tests.

Figure 5 compares the obtained results for the randomized models (blackened circles) to the actual starting model (circle).

It is clear that the obtained statistics for the modified vectors of lethal concentrations 50 are smaller than those of the real QSPR model, and for the most part one gets a $Q^2 < 0$. This ensures that a relationship (structure/lethal concentration 50) has been established each time.

3.5. External Validation

To ensure the effective predictive capacity of the model, we performed external validation on all 18 randomly selected compounds that are not a part of the test set.

A rigorous validation of the product model results in a large proportion of exact predictions given over the entire validation. The performance of the model is then measured by the regression coefficient R^2.

The obtained results show that the predicted values are close to the observed values.

The value of R^2 is 95.69, which confirms that the neuronal model adequately describes the relationship between lethal concentrations predicted and observed at 50.

pLC50pred = 0.798464 + 0.799547

pLC50 Obs $pLC50_{pred} = 0.0509872 + 0.993832\ pLC50_{Obs}$

S = 0.368047, R^2 = 70.6%, R^2 (adjusted) = 68.8%

S= 0.186772, R^2 = 93.5%, R^2 (adjusted) = 93.1%

The judgment of the quality of the models (MLR and ANN) was verified by calculating the RMSE; these statistical parameters are gathered below:

Table 4. Values of the statistical parameters for the validation set

	MLR	**ANN**
n	92	92
s	0.307	0.133
R^2	78.77	95.69
Q^2	76.04	94.91
Q^2ext	65.81	93.89
SDEC	0.292	0.13
SDEP	0.315	0.15
SDEPext	0.376	0.1589

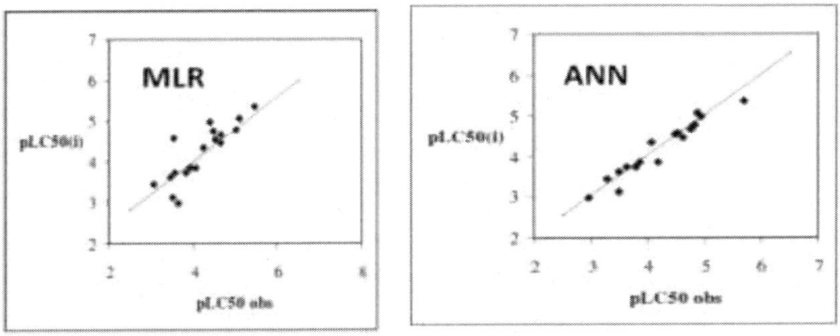

Figure 6. Graph of predicted pLĈ50 versus observed for validation.

General Conclusion

We applied the QSAR methodology to relate toxicity (LC50) to minnow (Pimephales promelas) and a series of potential organic pollutants in the aquatic environment. Two QSAR models were established using multilinear regression analysis and / or standard 3-layer neural networks (the inputs, a hidden layer and an output layer), with gradient backward learning algorithm (Levenberg-Marquard). The 92 basic data were randomly split into two disjoint sets, invariant for both models:

- a main set of 74 compounds used for the calculation and, possibly, tests the model;
- a set of 18 compounds for external prediction.

The size of the model (4 molecular descriptors) was fixed by maximizing KUBINYI's FIT function. The selection of the explanatory variables was carried out by genetic algorithm, in the MOBYDIGS version of TODESCHINI, by maximizing $Q2_{LOO}$. Statistics: R^2; σN and F's calculation established the relevance of the developed model.

The quality of the adjustment was verified by cross-validation by leave one-out. The value $Q^2 = 76.04$, clearly shows the quality of the adjustment. The randomization test shows that only the real vector of the observations leads to high values of the statistics R2 and Q2, which proves that the model obtained is not random with RMSE values (SDEC = 0.292, SDEP = 0.315, SDEPext = 0.376, Q2ext = 65.81).

This makes it possible to ensure, at the same time, the good predictive capacity of the model and its sufficient possibility of extension. Since the random selection of the set of tests can negatively influence the predictive capacity of the model, the method of extracting this set from the basic data must be redesigned.

Similarly, the limitations of the model must be defined more clearly, and the possible existence of outliers analyzed carefully. Finally, other methods that may prove more advantageous in terms of model accuracy and interpretation, and from the point of view of generalization capability, need to be tested.

References

[1] Lin, S. H. and Juang, R. S. 2009. "Adsorption of Phenol and Its Derivatives from Water Using Synthetic Resins and Low-Cost Natural Adsorbents: A Review". *Journal of Environmental Management,* 90:1336 - 1349.

[2] van Leeuwen C. J. and Vermeire T. G., *Risk Assessment Of Chemicals :An Introduction* (Ispra:Italy, Bilthoven:The Netherlands), 2007.

[3] Hodges et al., 2006. "Regional and cellular gene expression changes in human Huntington's disease brain, *Human Molecular Genetics, 15* no. 6(Feb. 2006).

[4] Todeschini, R. and Consonni, V., *Molecular Descriptors for Chemo-informatics*, (Wiley-VCH, 2009), 41.

[5] Kier, L. B. and Hall, L. H., *Molecular Connectivity in Chemistry and Drug Research*, (Academic Press, New York, 1975).

[6] HYPERCHEM Software (2002), Release 6.03 for Windows, Molecular Modeling System.

[7] Todeschini, R., V. Consonni, A. Mauri and M. Pavan, (2005), "Dragon Software for the calculation of molecular descriptors – Version 5.3 for Windows", Talete srl, Milano.

[8] Todeschini, R., D. Ballabio, V. Consonni, A. Mauri and M. Pavan, (2009), "Moby Digs Software for multilinear regression analysis and variable subset selection by genetic algorithm", Release 1.1 for Windows, Milano.

[9] Kubinyi, H. "Variable Selection in QSAR Studies. II. A Highly Efficient Combination of Systematic Search and Evolution". *Quantitative Structure-Activity Relationships*, 13: 285.

[10] Zupan, J. and J. Gasteiger, *Neural Networks for Chemists: An Introduction*, (VCH Publishers, Weinheim 1993).

Contents of Earlier Volumes

Advances in Health and Disease. Volume 13

Chapter 1 Dyslipidemia in Chronic Kidney Disease
Alicja E. Grzegorzewska

Chapter 2 Complex Pancreatic Trauma: Is There a Role for Autologous Islet Cell Transplants
D. J. Robinson, J. A. Logue, K. Oppong and S. A. White

Chapter 3 Dentofacial Changes After Adenotonsillectomy or Rapid Maxillary Expansion
Carolina M. Mordente, Bernardo Q. Souki, Paula L. Cheib, Kamila O. Machado and Letícia P. Franco

Chapter 4 Mouth Breathing and Dentofacial Growth Modification
Paula L. Cheib, Bernardo Q. Souki, Carolina M. Mordente, Kamila O. Machado and Letícia P. Franco

Chapter 5 Treatment of Multi-Drug Resistant Tuberculosis
Yamely Mendez, Daniel Arnaud, Ismael Garcia, Sara Surani, Francisco Eduardo Ochoa-Martinez, Jane Thomas and Salim Surani

Chapter 6 Clinicopathologic Features of Extranodal Marginal Zone Lymphoma of Mucosa-Associated Lymphoid Tissue (MALT Lymphoma) of the Dura
Daniel S. Socha and Richard A. Prayson

Chapter 7 Rapid Non-Invasive Diagnosis of Muscular Dystrophy at the Molecular Level
Kristina Zubow, Anatolij Zubow and Viktor Anatolievich Zubow

Advances in Health and Disease. Volume 12

Chapter 1 Adverse Effects of Oseltamivir in the Treatment of AH1N Virus Infections in Pediatric Populations
David Calderón Guzmán, Ernestina Hernández García, Hugo Juárez Olguín and Maribel Ortiz Herrera

Chapter 2 Foreign Body Aspiration as a Cause of Hemoptysis in Children
Giselle Cuestas

Chapter 3 Local Production of Estrogen and Breast Carcinogenesis
Danila Coradini

Chapter 4 Effect of Sildenafil on Neuroinflammatory Diseases
Sura Wanessa Santos Rocha, Letícia Nunes Campos, Ana Clara Santos Costa, Hélio Monteiro da Silva Filho and Ana Karolina Santana Nunes

Chapter 5 Effect of Sildenafil and Drug Homologues in the Treatment of Common Diseases
David Calderón Guzmán, Hugo Juárez Olguín, Maribel Ortiz Herrera, Fernanda Reyes Gonzalez and Gerardo Barragán Mejía

Chapter 6 My Life with Measles
C. John Clements

Chapter 7 Vasopressin and Schizophrenia
Bibiána Török and Dóra Zelena

Chapter 8 Flood Borne Dysentery
Kanaka Durga Devi Nelluri, Haritha Kondepati, Naveen Babu Kilaru and Navya Sree Thota

Chapter 9 The Role of Receptor Tyrosine Kinases in Bladder Cancer
Mehmet Alper Arslan and Sezgin Gunes

Advances in Health and Disease. Volume 11

Chapter 1 An Evaluation of Body Composition at a Cellular Level in Athletes: A Systematic Review
Priscila Custódio Martins, Mikael Seabra Moraes and Diego Augusto Santos Silva

Chapter 2 Diseases Associated with the Xenobiotic Receptor AhR Signaling Pathway and Lignans
Saimi Tokunaga

Chapter 3 Scrub Typhus Diagnostics: Culturing, Molecular and Serologic Detections
Hee Jung Lee, Seung Han Kim and Yoon-Won Kim

Chapter 4 Evidence Based Practice on Infection and Transmission of Disease in Residential Aged Care and Community Care Settings
Rasika Jayasekara

Chapter 5 Surgical Treatment of Choanal Atresia
Marco Berlucchi, Vittorio Rampinelli and Marco Ferrari

Chapter 6 Prevention of Diet-Induced Obesity in Rats by Administration of Peptides Derived from Marine Hydrobiont
Nataliia G. Raksha, Tetiana I. Halenova, Tetiana B. Vovk, Alena Y. Yurchenko, Iryna V. Nikoliaeva, Olexii M. Savchuk and Ludmila I. Ostapchenko

Chapter 7 Clinical and Microbiological Features of *Stenotrophomonas maltophilia* Infections in a Pediatric Tertiary-Care Hospital in South of Brazil
Luiza Souza Rodrigues, Jenifer Kogin Primon, Thaís Muniz Vasconcelos, Érika Medeiros dos Santos, Lavinia Nery Villa Stangler Arend, Guilherme Nardi Becker, Marinei Campos Ricieri and Libera Maria Dalla-Costa

Advances in Health and Disease. Volume 10

Chapter 1 Fertility Preservation Decision-Making
Dina M. Flink and Yvonne Kellar-Guenther

Chapter 2 Fertility Preservation: Indications, Procedures and Technological Advances
Sanghoon Lee and Seung-Yup Ku

Chapter 3 Understanding Why More Men Who Have Sex with Men (MSM) Are Not Using Pre-Exposure Prophylaxis (PrEP) Medication: Results from a Pilot Study
Hugh Klein and Thomas Alex Washington

Chapter 4 The Role of Flavonoids in Adipocyte Inflammation
Vânia Mayumi Nakajima, Cíntia Rabelo e Paiva Caria and Érica Martins F. Gotardo

Chapter 5 Molecular Mechanism Behind the Development of Chronic Kidney Disease
Rishila Ghosh and Pawan Kumar Kare

Advances in Health and Disease. Volume 9

Chapter 1 Advances in Health and Disease: Paracentesis in Medicine
Ana Clemente, Mario Romero, Diego Rincón, Jesus Millan, Rafael Bañares and Rita Garcia Martinez

Chapter 2 Tendinopathy: An Update from the Perspective of the Physiotherapist
Ana Gacimartín-García, Luis Prato and Luis Espejo-Antúnez

Chapter 3 Intrathecal Midazolam as an Analgesic in Chronic Back Pain
Jan Procházka

Chapter 4 Management of Intra-Articular Distal Radius Fractures with a Dorsal Locking Plate
Yoshihiro Abe and Hiromasa Wakita

Chapter 5 Complex Physiotherapeutic and Rehabilitation Programme Including Labor Activities in Patients After Distal Radius Fracture
Danelina Emilova Vacheva

Chapter 6 Evaluation of Symptomatic and Asymptomatic Meckel's Diverticulum
Anthony J. Ferrara and Sathyaprasad Burjonrappa

Chapter 7 Small Fish, Big Impact: Insights from Zebrafish on Human Diseases and Drug Discovery
Parth Thakkar, Chloe Shay and Yong Teng

Chapter 8 Zebrafish Model Used in Food Science and Technology: Antioxidant and Anti-Inflammatory Activities and Inhibition of Lipid Peroxidation
R. Vilcacundo, D. Barrio, L. Piñuel, P. Boeri, D. Morales, I. Angós, A. Pinto, A. Castro, W. Reyes and W. Carrillo

Chapter 9 Therapeutic Monitoring of Midazolam: An Approach to Adequate Sedation in Critically Ill Pediatric Patients
Carmen Flores Pérez, Janett Flores Pérez, Gabriela Peña Morales, Karen Delgado Vergara and Hugo Juárez Olguín

INDEX

A

Aedes aegypt, xi, 2, 8, 24, 28, 33, 124
Aedes albopictus (Stegomyia), xi, 2, 8
Africa, xiii, 4, 8, 9, 13, 22, 23, 24, 33, 94, 107
age, 22, 28, 33, 39, 43, 53, 58, 65, 78, 95, 143, 148, 149, 163, 164, 209, 210, 211, 213, 216, 217, 218
agencies, 12, 79, 84
aggregation, 147
AIDS, 32
air pollutants, 201
airways, 182
akinesia, 72
alanine, 212
albumin, 150, 152
Algeria, 229
algorithm, xxii, 230, 231, 232, 235, 240, 241, 242
alkaline phosphatase, 212
alopecia, xx, 188, 189, 190, 191, 192, 193, 196, 197
alopecia areata, xx, 188, 189, 190, 192, 193, 196, 197
ALT, 200, 205, 208, 212, 213, 220, 221
apoptosis, xvi, 6, 18, 145
aquatic toxicity, viii, 229, 230, 231, 232
arbovirus infection, 22
Arboviruses, 10, 99, 138
Argentina, xiv, 4, 207, 216
arousal, 158
arrest, 16
artery, 179, 180
arthralgia, 11, 22, 23, 28, 30, 51, 52, 57, 59, 66
arthritis, 190
arthrogryposis, 71
arthropod-borne virus (arbovirus), 8, 22, 92, 102, 106, 113
Artificial Neural Networks, 233, 235
avoidance behavior, 30
awareness, 23, 79, 90

C

calcifications, xvi, 6, 19, 37, 39, 43, 52, 64, 71, 72
calcium, 149, 152
Cambodia, 23

campaigns, 27
cancer, 166, 190, 222, 223, 224, 225
candidates, 10, 13, 95, 98, 107, 172
carcinogen, 201
caregivers, 43, 58, 164
Caribbean, 9, 27, 46
carpal tunnel syndrome, 159
CDC, xiv, 5, 11, 27, 30, 32, 36, 41, 44, 46, 49, 50, 51, 55, 59, 60, 64, 65, 66, 70, 79, 80, 81, 82, 83, 85, 87, 89, 92, 99, 111, 131
Central African Republic, xiii, 3
central nervous system, 19
central nervous system (CNS), 19
cephalgia, 9
cerebrospinal fluid, 18
cerebrovascular complications, 18
challenges, 13, 69, 73, 88, 91, 95, 97, 98, 100, 104, 112, 125, 135
chemical, xxii, 201, 206, 207, 214, 215, 230, 231, 232
chemical industry, 215
chemicals, x, xxi, 199, 201, 204, 213, 222, 230, 231
chemotherapy, xviii, 140, 154, 159, 160, 169, 170, 192, 194, 195
Chicago, 170, 171
Chikungunya Virus (CHIKV), xv, 5, 8, 24, 33, 63, 92
childhood, 95, 204, 222, 224, 225
childhood cancer, 222
children, x, xxi, 36, 41, 42, 50, 56, 57, 59, 63, 71, 74, 78, 81, 85, 90, 128, 199, 204, 205, 206, 207, 208, 209, 210, 211, 212, 213, 214, 215, 216, 217, 218, 219, 220, 221, 224, 225, 226, 227
cough, 162, 207, 208, 213, 216, 217, 218
creatinine, 148, 152, 205, 210, 211, 221
cyclophosphamide, 160, 172, 173, 174

D

damages, iv, 16
data set, 232
database, 41, 181, 182
deaths, xvii, 6, 56
deciliter, 150
defects, 14, 19, 21, 32, 37, 39, 41, 42, 46, 49, 51, 91
deficiency, 157, 158
dehydration, 156
demyelinating disease, 179
dendritic cell, xiv, 4
dengue, x, xiv, xvii, 2, 5, 7, 23, 63, 74, 77, 85, 94, 95, 99, 113, 138
dengue fever, 23
Dengue Virus (DENV), xv, 5, 8, 22, 33, 62, 63, 86, 92, 94
dependent variable, 233
destruction, 16, 37, 71, 145, 153, 157, 192
detectable, 64, 221
detection, 35, 50, 55, 63, 68, 73, 79
detoxification, 212, 219
developed countries, 76, 92
developing brain, 39
diagnostic criteria, xviii, 139, 155, 165
diarrhea, 162, 208, 218
differential diagnosis, xv, 5, 63
diffusion, 179

F

false negative, 153
families, 20, 42, 46, 78, 214
family planning, 84, 86, 132
fat, 192
FDA, 90, 93, 191, 194
fear, 75
fears, 74
female rat, 143
fertility, 59

fetal demise, 30
fetal development, 11, 16, 21
fetal growth, 52
fetus, xvi, 6, 8, 13, 15, 16, 21, 37, 45, 80, 96, 123
fever, x, xv, xviii, 2, 5, 7, 9, 11, 22, 23, 28, 30, 51, 52, 57, 59, 66, 68, 94
fibroblasts, 14, 16
fibrosis, 191
Fiji, xiii, 4
financial, 221
fish, 231
fixation, 135
Flaviviridae, ix, x, 1, 8
Flavivirus, ix, x, 1, 8, 13, 14, 29, 47, 62, 70, 86, 94, 95, 97, 98
fluid, xii, 3, 60
fluorescence, 158
follicles, 191
Food and Drug Administration, 90, 162, 191
force, 34, 38
formation, 16, 157, 218
fractures, 157
fragments, 141
free radicals, 224
funding, 75, 86
fusion, 16, 193, 194

G

Gabon, xi, xiii, 2, 3
gait, 217
ganglion, 185
gene expression, 19, 145, 167, 190, 242
genes, 15, 17, 19, 20, 146, 218
genetic alteration, 144
genetic background, 21
genetic disorders, 42
genetic factors, 143
genetics, 100, 169
genome, xi, xvi, 2, 6, 13
genomic stability, xxi, 200
genre, xi, 2
genus, ix, x, xv, 1, 5, 8, 13, 23
Georgia, 46, 91, 117
gestation, 15, 56, 71, 87
gestational age, 38, 45, 48, 51, 72
glaucoma, 192
glia, 19
global warming, 69
glycosylation, 13
governments, xiii, 4, 74
grades, 90, 191
graph, 234, 235, 236
growth, x, xiii, xxi, 4, 14, 17, 34, 43, 58, 144, 148, 166, 190, 192, 195, 197, 199, 204
growth factor, 144, 148
Guatemala, xiii, xvi, 4, 6, 56
guidance, 45, 52, 55, 65, 67, 70, 82, 83, 89, 93
guidelines, xix, 44, 51, 56, 59, 62, 64, 81, 122, 136, 140, 164, 168, 172
Guillain-Barré syndrome, xvi, 6, 7, 8, 108, 116

H

headache, xv, 5, 11, 28, 158
health, x, xvii, xxi, 6, 12, 24, 28, 32, 33, 35, 42, 45, 47, 51, 56, 57, 59, 60, 62, 64, 65, 66, 73, 74, 76, 77, 78, 79, 80, 85, 87, 92, 100, 199, 201, 204, 211, 213, 215, 218, 221, 222, 223, 224, 225, 226
health care, 35, 47, 51, 56, 60, 64, 65, 66, 74, 79, 85, 88, 92
health care system, 67
health effects, xxi, 199, 201, 204, 215, 221, 222, 223, 224, 226
health risks, 211, 213
health services, 75, 78
hearing impairment, xix, 178

hearing loss, 40, 179, 180, 181, 182, 183, 184, 185, 186
heart failure, 159
hematocrit, 205, 210, 211, 218, 221
hematopoietic system, 141
hemisphere, xi, 2
hemoglobin, 149, 205, 209, 210, 211, 218, 221
hemorrhage, 63
hepatic injury, 220
herbal medicine, 99
heterogeneity, 147
high school, 89
histocompatibility antigens, 144
history, 12, 20, 51, 62, 80, 102, 122, 184
HIV, 32, 36, 92, 111
HIV/AIDS, 32
HLA, 148
HLA antigens, 148
homes, 29
Honduras, xvi, 6, 56
hospitalization, 28
host, xxi, 17, 21, 34, 69, 100, 167, 180, 190, 200, 202, 204
hot spots, 47
human, xiii, 3, 8, 9, 14, 15, 17, 18, 20, 23, 24, 27, 33, 35, 61, 64, 77, 103, 104, 105, 130, 135, 166, 167, 189, 201, 227, 233, 242
human brain, 20, 105, 233
human exposure, 201
human health, 33, 35
human right, 130
human rights, 130
hybrid, x, xxii, 230
Hybrid GA/ANN model, 230
hydrocephalus, xvi, 6, 71
hydroquinone, 202
hyperbaric oxygen therapy, ix, xx, 178, 179, 184, 185, 186
hypercalcemia, xviii, 140, 155, 157
hyperemia, 68
hypereosinophilic syndrome, xx, 188, 189
139, 242

J

Janus Kinase (JAK), xx, 188, 189, 190, 191, 192, 196, 197
Japanese Encephalitis Virus (JEV), 8
joint pain, 218
joints, 208, 218, 220
Jordan, 109, 110, 119, 120
jurisdiction, 27
Jurisdictions, 49, 92

M

macromolecules, 212, 219
macrophages, 14, 16, 103
madarosis, xx, 188, 189, 192, 193
magnetic resonance, xviii, 73, 140, 152, 153, 154, 169
magnetic resonance imaging, 73, 152, 153, 154, 169
magnitude, 24, 68
majority, 29, 73, 147
malabsorption, 159
mental retardation, 20, 40
mesenchymal stem cells, 16
messages, 45, 89
messenger RNA, 95
meta-analysis, 175, 184, 223
metabolic pathways, 202
metabolism, xxi, 200, 202, 203, 212, 219, 224
metabolites, 202, 204, 224
metabolized, 202
metals, xxi, 229
methodology, 65, 240
methylation, 219
Mexico, xiii, xvi, 4, 6, 25, 48, 56, 86
Miami, 46

mice, xvi, 6, 20, 137
microcephaly, xiii, xvi, 3, 6, 7, 9, 11, 14, 18, 19, 21, 24, 25, 30, 31, 32, 35, 37, 38, 39, 41, 44, 46, 52, 55, 60, 63, 64, 66, 70, 71, 72, 73, 75, 78, 87, 100, 106, 107, 108, 111, 114, 115, 116, 117, 120, 123, 128, 129, 138
microcirculation, 158
Middle East, 68
migration, 19, 71
miscarriage, 9
misconceptions, 84
mitosis, xvi, 6
model system, 61
models, 10, 13, 21, 34, 97, 231, 233, 238, 239, 240
molecular biology, xix, 140, 165
molecular weight, 148
molecules, 98, 153, 231
monoclonal antibody, 162
morbidity, 84, 100, 192
morphology, 69
mosquito bites, 30, 32, 55, 76, 79, 81, 86, 99
mosquitoes, xi, xv, xvii, 2, 5, 7, 8, 9, 12, 23, 27, 33, 69, 75, 77, 81, 85, 88, 132
motor neurons, 72
MRI, 73, 152, 153, 154, 155
mRNA, 95
mucosa, 158
mucous membrane, 157
mucous membranes, 157
mucus, 60
multiple myeloma, ix, xviii, xix, 140, 141, 142, 154, 165, 166, 167, 168, 169, 170, 171, 172, 173, 174, 175, 176, 223
mutations, 141, 146, 150, 190, 194, 202
myalgia, 11, 23, 28
myelin, 20
myelofibrosis, x, xx, 187, 188, 190, 191, 194
myeloproliferative disorders, 189

P

population, xv, 5, 24, 26, 29, 34, 35, 46, 61, 72, 76, 78, 85, 87, 88, 96, 99, 143, 191, 201, 214, 222, 224
population growth, 99
population size, 34
Portugal, 208, 217
positron, 152, 153, 169
positron emission tomography, 152, 153, 169
precursor cells, 18
prednisone, 159, 161, 174, 175
pregnancy, vii, xii, xvi, xviii, 1, 3, 6, 7, 8, 11, 14, 15, 25, 31, 32, 35, 38, 39, 41, 44, 45, 50, 51, 52, 55, 57, 58, 60, 61, 63, 64, 65, 70, 74, 78, 79, 82, 84, 85, 87, 89, 95, 97, 98, 103, 104, 111, 113, 114, 115, 116, 117, 118, 119, 122, 123, 124, 126, 127, 130, 131, 133, 134, 137, 138, 216, 224
preparation, iv, 79, 170
preparedness, 75, 90
preservation, 195
President, 75

R

radiation, 144, 146
Ramadan, 222
rash, xv, 5, 11, 22, 23, 25, 27, 30, 37, 38, 39, 51, 52, 57, 59, 66, 68, 162
RBC, 200, 205, 208, 209, 210, 221
reactions, 22, 97, 189, 191
reactive oxygen, 224
reactivity, 62, 206, 215
reading, 13
reality, 86
recall, 93
receptor, 19, 99, 145
receptors, 190

recognition, 36, 65, 79
recombination, 13
recommendations, iv, 51, 62, 64, 80, 81, 84, 86, 87, 131, 225
reconstruction, 145
resistance, 146, 158, 202
resource allocation, 75
resources, 12, 33, 61, 74, 78, 88, 91, 122
response, 11, 13, 15, 16, 26, 28, 32, 35, 41, 50, 54, 65, 67, 70, 74, 77, 86, 88, 90, 97, 153, 159, 161, 163, 164, 168, 171, 176, 191, 225
retinoblastoma, 146
rheumatoid arthritis, 190
rhinitis, 207, 216
rhythm, 158
ribonucleic acid, ix, x, xv, 1, 5, 8, 95
ribonucleic acid (RNA), ix, x, xiii, xv, 1, 4, 5, 8, 18, 38, 53, 60, 63, 69, 92, 95, 98, 219, 236
ribonucleic acid (RNA) virus, x, 1, 8
rights, iv, 77, 78, 130
risk, x, xi, xv, xvii, xix, xxi, 2, 5, 7, 11, 16, 22, 30, 32, 39, 45, 49, 52, 57, 59, 63, 66, 69, 74, 75, 78, 80, 81, 83, 84, 85, 87, 89, 93, 94, 96, 100, 112, 132, 140, 142, 149, 150, 151, 155, 160, 165, 168, 191, 199, 202, 206, 214, 215, 217, 223, 224, 230
risk assessment, 224, 230
risk factors, x, xxi, 100, 142, 199
risks, 14, 26, 53, 55, 60, 79, 80, 85, 87, 93, 143, 147, 162, 163, 164, 218, 222, 225, 230
RNA, x, xiii, 1, 4, 8, 18, 38, 53, 60, 63, 70, 92, 95, 98, 219, 236
rodents, xii, 2
root, 20
routes, xii, 3, 8, 31, 32, 63, 107
rubella, xv, 5, 94
ruxolitinib, vii, x, xx, 187, 188, 189, 190, 191, 192, 193, 194, 196, 197

S

statistics, 238, 241
stem cells, 18, 105, 123
steroids, 179, 181
stock, xiii, 4
storage, 135
storms, 81
stratification, 165
stress, 156
structural characteristics, xi, 2
structural protein, 98
structure, x, 10, 141, 231, 232, 236, 239
subcutaneous tissue, 158
subgroups, 61, 146
subjective experience, 195
Substituted Benzenes, viii, x, xxii, 229, 230
success rate, 182, 183
Sudden sensorineural hearing loss, ix, xix, 177, 178, 184, 185, 186
Sun, 194
suppression, 141, 154
surveillance, 9, 22, 27, 38, 41, 42, 44, 45, 49, 61, 67, 68, 88, 89
survival, 148, 151, 154, 161, 167, 168, 171, 172, 175
survival rate, 151
survivors, 73
susceptibility, xxi, 157, 199, 204, 224
symptoms, xv, xvii, xviii, 5, 7, 8, 12, 28, 30, 40, 51, 52, 66, 71, 93, 110, 140, 155, 156, 157, 178, 206, 207, 208, 213, 214, 215, 216, 217, 218, 220, 221, 223, 226
synaptogenesis, 8
syndrome, xvi, xx, 6, 7, 8, 19, 39, 70, 94, 108, 128, 158, 159, 188, 189
synthesis, xxi, 230
syphilis, 36

T

testing, x, xxii, 11, 17, 26, 27, 30, 39, 45, 50, 51, 55, 56, 57, 58, 60, 62, 64, 65, 66, 70, 88, 93, 97, 230
testis, 98
Thailand, xiii, 3
Theoretical Molecular Descriptors, 230
therapeutic approaches, 142
therapeutic interventions, 62
therapeutic targets, 167
therapeutics, 22, 98
therapy, ix, xv, xvii, xix, xx, 5, 7, 38, 76, 99, 140, 148, 154, 159, 161, 164, 170, 171, 172, 173, 174, 175, 178, 179, 181, 182, 183, 184, 185, 186, 189, 193, 195
threats, 99
thrombocytopenia, 9, 28, 191, 219
time lags, 25
time series, 25
time use, 68

W

Washington, 122, 247
water, xv, 5, 30, 80, 201
weakness, 11
web, 214
weight loss, 218
well-being, 77
West Africa, 9, 13
West Nile Virus (WNV), 8
wheezing, 206, 207, 208, 215, 216, 217, 218, 220, 227
white blood cells, 218
white matter, xvi, 6
WHO, xiii, 4, 11, 24, 31, 43, 46, 54, 60, 66, 74, 84, 86, 93, 95, 97, 116
wildlife, 13
windows, 30
withdrawal, 84
workers, 222
World Health Organization, xiii, 4, 9
World Health Organization (WHO), xiii, 4, 9
worldwide, 10, 12, 36, 60, 76, 99, 107
worry, 123

Y

yellow fever, x, 2, 22, 23, 77, 94, 106, 113, 135
Yellow Fever Virus (YFV), xv, 5, 8, 94

Z

Zika Virus (ZIKV), vii, ix, x, xiii, xiv, 1, 3, 5, 7, 8, 9, 10, 13, 14, 15, 17, 18, 19, 21, 22, 23, 24, 26, 27, 30, 31, 32, 33, 35, 36, 38, 39, 41, 42, 43, 44, 45, 49, 50, 51, 54, 55, 57, 58, 59, 60, 62, 63, 64, 65, 66, 69, 70, 71, 72, 75, 77, 79, 80, 81, 82, 83, 84, 85, 86, 87, 89, 92, 93, 95, 96, 97, 99, 101, 102, 103, 104, 105, 106, 107, 108, 109, 110, 111, 112, 113, 114, 115, 116, 117, 118, 119, 120, 121, 122, 123, 124, 125, 126, 127, 128, 129, 130, 131, 132, 133, 134, 135, 136, 137, 138